little book of sex

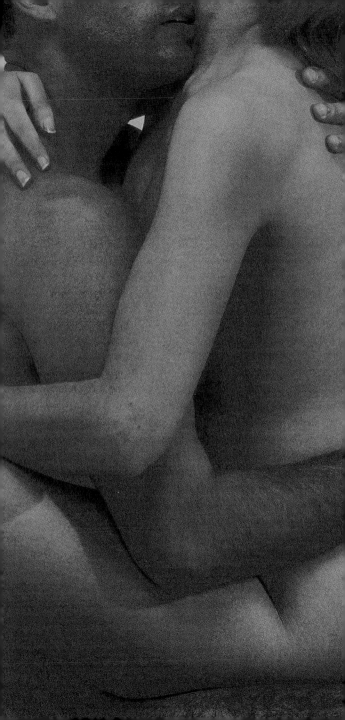

little book
of sex

Anne Hooper

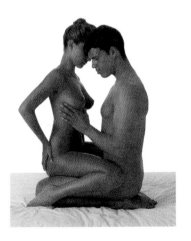

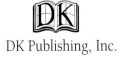

DK Publishing, Inc.

LONDON, NEW YORK, MUNICH,
MELBOURNE, DELHI

Senior Editor Salima Hirani
US Senior Editor Jennifer Williams
Project Editor Jane Sarluis
Art Editors Kelly Meyer, Iona Hoyle
US Assistant Editor John Searcy
DTP Designer Julian Dams

Managing Editors Maxine Lewis, Jemima Dunne
Managing Art Editor Heather McCarry
Senior Art Editor Helen Spencer

Production Controller Sarah Sherlock
Brand Manager Lynne Brown

Publishing Director Corinne Roberts
Art Director Carole Ash

First American Edition 2005
05 06 07 08 09 10 9 8 7 6 5 4 3 2 1

Published in the United States in 2005 by DK Publishing, Inc.
375 Hudson Street, New York, New York 10014
A Penguin Company

Cataloging-in-Publication data is available from
the Library of Congress
ISBN 0 7566 1036 2

Color reproduction by Media Development Printing Ltd,
United Kingdom
Printed and bound by Star Standard,
Singapore

See our complete product line at

www.dk.com

Contents

What's Inside

Each section of the book contains visual aids designed to help you process the information quickly and easily. Features include symbols that highlight important, interesting, or technical points, step-by-step boxes, and summary lists for each chapter.

Key to Symbols

Very Important Point: this symbol points out information that you really need to know before continuing.

Getting Technical: you'll need to slow down and read carefully when you see this symbol.

Inside Scoop: helpful tips from the author's personal experience are indicated by this symbol.

Complete No-No: this symbol is a warning and advises you when not to do something.

Concise text: each paragraph is self-contained and comes with its own heading.

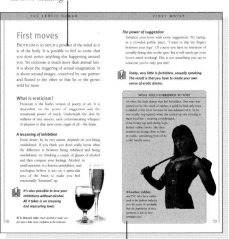

Yellow Boxes: for additional or simply interesting information, check out the colored boxes.

Instruction boxes: *these guide you through difficult or challenging activities, often step by step.*

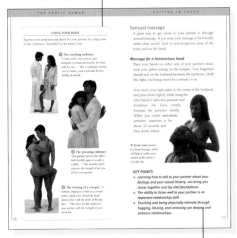

Key Points: *each chapter ends on a list of bulleted points that sum up the key issues discussed.*

Author Biography

Anne Hooper is the international best-selling author of over 35 books that have been translated into 15 languages. A sex and marriage counselor for 20 years, she was part of the movement that pioneered sex therapy in the US and Britain in the 1970s. She founded the Women's Sexuality Workshop, which offered help to women unable to climax, and gave sex and relationship advice to radio call-ins for two decades. She has also appeared on television and radio all over the US, Australia, and New Zealand.

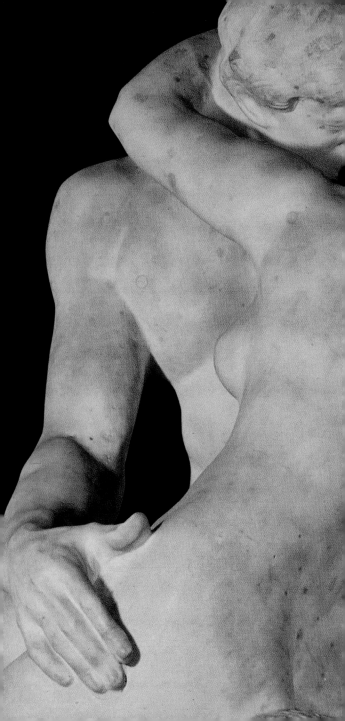

Part One

The Erotic Human

Some of the most exciting times in a new relationship are the precious moments between love's first appearance and its consummation. The transformation from an emotional and spiritual relationship to a sexual one is an occasion to prepare for some wonderful lovemaking. Whether you are a sexual novice or an experienced lover, use this time to build something special. It may not be fashionable to take things slowly, but by preparing yourself for sex (this includes making sure that sex is safe) you can greatly enhance the quality of your experience.

In this part...

- **Getting in touch**
- **First moves**
- **What men expect**
- **What women expect**
- **First sex**
- **Journey to the interior**

Getting in touch

THE KEYS TO good sex are plenty of sensual touch combined with good communication. So start your relationship not only by exploring each other's body but by discovering the pleasure, romance, and excitement of talking – about, during, and after sex.

Tempting talk

You're feeling great about your partner. Mutual physical attraction has flowered into an emotional connection, and you're delighted to find that everything about your lover drives you wild. Don't keep these feelings to yourself. Talking gets you into the habit of being open and makes your partner feel wonderful.

Simple sex talk

Learn about your partner's sexuality – what turns them on and off and what makes them comfortable and uncomfortable – before you jump into bed. A good way to do this is by sharing your **sexual biographies**.

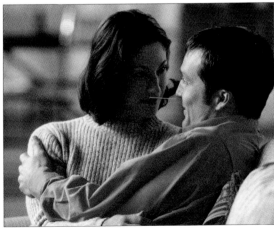

■ **Talking to your partner** *about sex is a vital part of your relationship, particularly when you are getting to know somebody new.*

Your sexual biography is composed of all the thoughts, feelings, and experiences that have contributed to your sexuality.

A SEXUAL BIOGRAPHY

Your sexual biography consists of:

- *Your family background – the cultural and religious attitudes of your parents, their attitude toward nudity, how they related to one another, whether you ever "caught them at it" (and if so, how you reacted), and what they taught you about sex*

- *Your formal sex education*

- *Your informal sex education – what you picked up from siblings, friends, and school*

- *When you first masturbated, and what your early fantasies were*

- *Your earliest sexual experience with either gender*

- *Your previous partners, if you have been sexually active*

Simply expressing your feelings

Exposing your inner feelings can be difficult. Try to use phrases such as "I feel this…" or "I sense that…" Avoid using "you" as it can seem accusatory and impersonal.

Practicing in front of a mirror is a useful exercise. You get accustomed to saying and hearing yourself say things you might not have thought possible.

 Be aware of which phrases make you look uncomfortable. Keep practicing these words until you are less self-conscious.

Don't forget to listen

Conversations have two sides, so you need to listen as well as talk. Being a good listener is a simple, but invaluable, asset.

 Don't ever be fooled into thinking that listening is a passive, effortless state.

Good listening techniques

You should regularly practice these listening techniques:

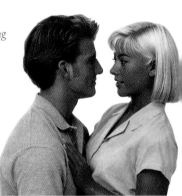

- *Concentrate on what your partner is saying*
- *Give feedback*
- *Don't interrupt*
- *Encourage your partner to elaborate*

■ **Take the time** *to listen to your partner. Lending a sympathetic ear is good for your relationship.*

Tempting touch

Build up to sex in little ways and use simple touch to do so. When you are first trying to make an impression, touch can be a subtle signal of desire and attraction. It is a powerful tool to be used in the initial mating dance.

Good timing for simple touch

Touching is great, but not appropriate to every situation. For example, avoid intimate contact with work colleagues. Touching your partner at the wrong time may also be off-putting and could set back your relationship.

 Be sensitive about the possible squeamishness of others. Do not be too demonstrative in front of parents, children, or exes.

Gauge the emotional temperature

You should also be sensitive about your timing within the relationship. Every relationship is unique, and therefore there are no hard-and-fast rules about when or what sort of touching is okay.

Go slowly and start with innocuous touches. A touch on the knee to emphasize a point or a grateful squeeze of the shoulder can speak volumes about your feelings.

 Try to recognize your partner's signals and respond accordingly. Does she lean close to you, or does he gaze intently into your eyes?

Seize the opportunity

Once you've got the green light, make the most of it. Angle your body to face your partner, lean close, and rest one arm on the back of the sofa so that your fingers can teasingly caress his shoulder. Let your breath tickle her ear. Hold hands, hug, and kiss. Go somewhere you can slow dance together.

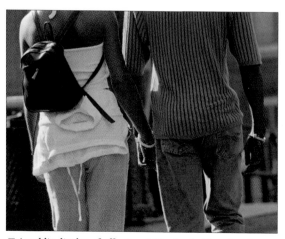

■ **A public display of affection:** *holding hands while walking down the street is a sign of intimacy between you and your partner.*

Simple kissing and hugging

Kissing is one of the most intimate, meaningful contacts that you can have with another person. Some cultures explicitly acknowledge the sanctity of this mingling of breaths and therefore of life forces. Many prostitutes will not kiss their clients on the mouth, reserving this most intimate of contacts for their personal relationships.

Ancient advice on touch

The **Kama Sutra**, the ancient Indian manual of sexual and erotic wisdom, focuses on heavy **petting**.

Petting involves physically touching, caressing, hugging, and kissing in a sexual or erotic manner. It can also lead to sexual intercourse.

In the 2,000-year-old *Kama Sutra*, making love is elevated to an art form. From embracing and caressing to kissing and biting, each erotic element has been explored and described in lingering detail, offering modern lovers a wealth of ideas on which to draw.

■ **Kissing and caressing** *are an integral part of heavy petting, whether or not this leads to intercourse.*

Using your nails

The Kama Sutra also details the erotic uses of scratching. Use your nails to gently scrape your partner's skin – hard enough to leave a faint mark, but not so hard that the skin is broken. Draw your nails slowly down the fleshy areas of the back, waist, and buttocks.

USING YOUR LIPS

The *Kama Sutra* lists dozens of kisses, ranging from the tentative to the passionate. By exploring these options you can express affection as well as lust and desire.

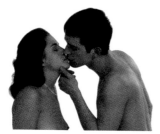

1 **The turned kiss:** *"One of them turns up the face of the other by holding the head and chin, and then kissing."* This gentle kiss expresses feelings of tenderness.

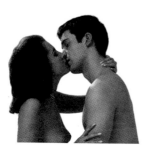

2 **The bent kiss:** *"The heads of two lovers are bent towards each other."* This is a natural angle for deep, passionate kissing.

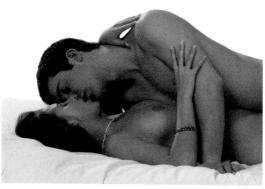

3 **The clasping kiss:** *"Take both the lips of the other in your own… if one of you touches the teeth, the tongue, and the palate of the other with your tongue, it is called the fighting of the tongue."*

USING YOUR BODY

Express your attraction and desire for your partner by using some of the "embraces" described in the *Kama Sutra*.

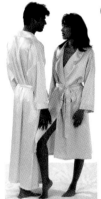

1 The touching embrace:
"A man, under some pretext, goes alongside a woman and touches her body with his own…" This is a playful, teasing sort of contact, used to provoke the first feelings of arousal.

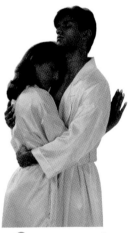

2 The pressing embrace:
"One partner presses the other's body forcibly against a wall or a pillar…" This raunchy clinch expresses the strength of lust you feel for your partner.

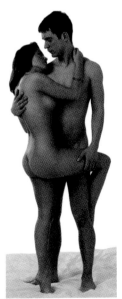

3 The twining of a creeper: *"A woman, clinging to a man as a creeper twines round a tree, bends his head down to hers with the desire of kissing him…"* This move forcibly impresses your partner with the strength of your attraction.

Sensual massage

A great way to get closer to your partner is through sensual massage. If you want your massage to be friendly rather than sexual, stick to nonerogenous areas of the body, such as the head.

Massage for a harmonious head

Place your hands on either side of your partner's head, with your palms resting on the temples. Your fingertips should rest on the forehead between the eyebrows. Hold this light, enclosing touch for a minute or so.

Now move your right palm to the center of the forehead, and press down lightly, while using the other hand to add extra pressure and distribute the force evenly. Increase the pressure slowly. When you reach maximum pressure, maintain it for about 10 seconds and then slowly release.

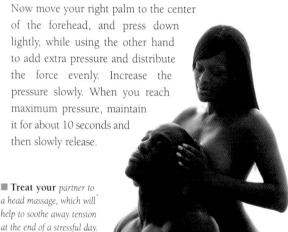

■ **Treat your** *partner to a head massage, which will help to soothe away tension at the end of a stressful day.*

KEY POINTS

- *Learning how to talk to your partner about your feelings and your sexual history can bring you closer together and lay vital foundations.*
- *The ability to listen well to your partner is an important relationship skill.*
- *Touching and being physically intimate through hugging, kissing, and caressing can deepen and enhance relationships.*

First moves

EROTICISM IS AS MUCH a product of the mind as it is of the body. It is possible to feel so erotic that you do not notice anything else happening around you. Yet eroticism is much more than animal lust. It is about the triggering of your sexual imagination. It is about sensual images, conceived by one partner and transmitted to the other so that he or she grows wild for more.

What is eroticism?

Eroticism is the body's version of poetry or art. It is dependent on the power of suggestion and the sensational power of touch. Underneath the skin lie millions of tiny sensors, each communicating whispers of pleasure to that most erotic organ of all – the brain.

A lessening of inhibition

Erotic desire, by its very nature, depends on your being uninhibited. If you think you don't really know what the difference is between being inhibited and being uninhibited, try drinking a couple of glasses of alcohol and then compare your feelings. Alcohol, in small amounts, is a known uninhibitor, and **sexologists** believe it acts on a particular area of the brain to make you feel emotionally "loosened" up.

It's also possible to lose your inhibitions without alcohol. All it takes is an arousing and reassuring lover.

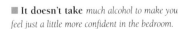
■ **It doesn't take** *much alcohol to make you feel just a little more confident in the bedroom.*

The power of suggestion

Tantalize your lover with erotic suggestions. Try saying, in a crowded public place, "I want to slip my fingers between your legs." Naturally, you have no intention of actually doing this on the spot. But it will surely get your lover's mind working! Of course, this is not something you say to someone you've only just met!

Today, very little is forbidden, sexually speaking. The result is that you have to create your own sense of erotic drama.

WHAT FEELS FORBIDDEN TO YOU?

It's often the little things that feel forbidden. One man was turned on by the smell of rubber, a quirk he had only once confided to his lover because he was ashamed of it. So he was totally unprepared when she turned up one evening at their local bar – wearing a rubberized, close-fitting top and slinky, high-heeled rubber boots. She then insisted on sitting close to him in public, tantalizing him until he could hardly move.

■ **Leather, rubber,**
and PVC have been widely used in the fashion industry over the years. It's probable that the popularity of these garments is due to their forbidden feel.

Who creates eroticism – him or her?

There are people who can't help being erotic, and people who only find eroticism by accident. Some people say eroticism differs between the sexes; others say that gender doesn't enter into it.

Him – eroticism through sexual imagination

Some sexologists have proposed a controversial theory suggesting that men have a more sexual imagination than women. According to these sex scientists, this is because men possess a greater amount of the hormone **testosterone** than women.

Her – eroticism through perception

While a man may or may not rely more on his imagination, a woman certainly relies on her powers of perception. Perception is the finely honed instinct of reading and comprehending unspoken messages, understanding what is between the lines, and interpreting body language.

The strength of simple subtlety

If you are a woman, subtlety can be about:

- *turning in profile so that he can see the silhouette of your beautiful body*

- *standing back-to-back at a party and touching "by accident."*

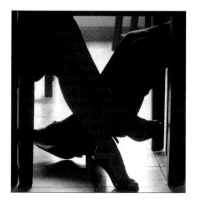

■ **When out in public** *the occasional "accidental" touch – unnoticed by anyone but him – can be highly effective in creating an erotic tension.*

If you are a man, subtlety is about:

- *staring at her across a crowded room, and when she notices you, staring a beat longer before glancing away*

- *lazily stroking her while in conversation with another*

- *taking her bare arm while side-by-side in the movie theater, and stroking it on the inside with your fingernails.*

The dynamics of being direct

There are some individuals who wouldn't recognize subtlety if it slapped them across the face. But be direct with them, and suddenly all rockets are firing.

Simple, direct erotic action might consist of:

- *saying, "You're gorgeous. Come and have dinner with me tonight?"*

- *taking your partner in your arms underneath a lamp post, and kissing him unexpectedly and skillfully*

- *letting an impromptu kiss evolve of its own accord*

- *passionately kissing your partner when you get back to his or her place and, provided you aren't rejected, going on from there.*

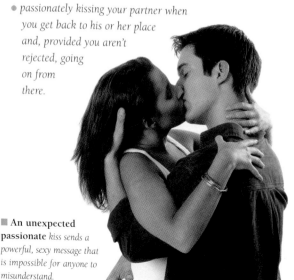

■ **An unexpected passionate** kiss sends a powerful, sexy message that is impossible for anyone to misunderstand.

21

Setting the scene

Imagine a room with dim but rosy lighting, Eastern drapes, the scent of incense in the background, and a four-poster bed draped with silken fringes and satin sheets. Or what about a room with night-black walls, silken ropes hanging from sturdy hooks, and an array of stainless-steel sex toys? Which of the two scenes feels more comfortable? What ideas form in your imagination? When it comes to eroticism, the appearance and ambiance of your bedroom is very important.

Make the bedroom sexy

Start by identifying the themes that appeal to your particular brand of eroticism. Do you love the idea of being a **virgin** who is "taken" on her bed by a rampaging crusader? All-white muslin drapes and lacy pillowcases would set the scene. Or what about a gothic look – a four-poster bed, scarlet and black drapes, and massive cathedral candles? Or how about classic *Kama Sutra* terrain? Sprinkle fresh flowers and herbs across the sheets so that every time you roll, fresh scents rise from underneath your heated bodies. If urgency is your theme, perhaps the living room will be sexier for you than the bedroom. Think about it.

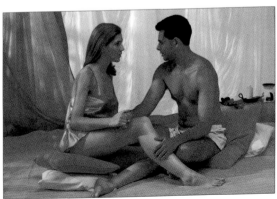

■ **As with any** home decor, the bedroom's colors, motifs, and furnishings should make you feel a certain way. So choose something erotic for this room.

Talking dirty

Some men and women are immensely turned on by talking dirty. This is great, provided you feel comfortable with it. But a lot of people grow up thinking that virtually any of the words concerning sex, even perfectly straightforward ones, such as "masturbation," are negative. And they probably learned this as children. These people may find it very difficult to talk dirty.

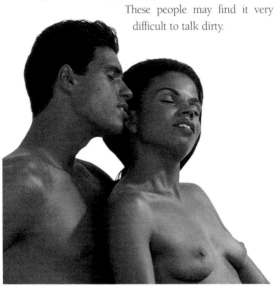

■ **Once you are comfortable** *with so-called dirty words, you will be free to use them in the bedroom, if you so desire. It may have a great effect.*

A famous sex therapy technique for people who are sexually shy consists of watching an actor reading aloud a list of dirty words. After the 100th word or so people tend to become desensitized.

Perfecting your dirty talk

To become more comfortable with "talking dirty" to your partner, try this **desensitization technique** at home. Draw up a checklist of "loaded" words and then say them out loud in front of a mirror. When you can say them without cringing, you are ready to talk dirty.

23

Simple sensual touch

If you are hungry for sex, or have been longing for sexual connection for months, you will probably be in a hurry. This is normal and understandable for you, but it may not always be appropriate for your partner. It's worth knowing that one of the best sex tips is to remember to simply slow down.

Remember that your fingers are your greatest asset. The lover who is a maestro of finger-tipping is the lover everyone wants to keep!

Sensual strokes

Lie down side-by-side with your partner and try the following techniques.

- *run the tips of your fingers unhurriedly across each other's skin*
- *walk your fingers along your partner's body*
- *swirl your fingertips in opposite directions*
- *use your fingernails only.*

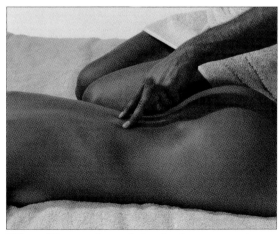

■ **Try walking your fingers** *slowly and gently up your partner's spine. Start at the base, work up to the nape of the neck, then work down again.*

Slow-motion massage

The skin experiences slow, drawn-out touch as endless erotic sensation. This sensation becomes so mind-bending that you never want it to cease. When it comes to erotic touch, the emphasis is always on slowing things down.

 Don't speed up! When someone speeds up touch, it is hard to relax and difficult not to feel pressured.

Two bodies together

The first time one naked body slithers across another is a uniquely wonderful sensation. Never underestimate it.

The simple pleasures of erotic touch include:

- *the texture of your partner's skin*

- *the softness or firmness of your partner's flesh*

- *the way in which your partner moves against your body*

- *your partner's* **genitals** *against your genitals.*

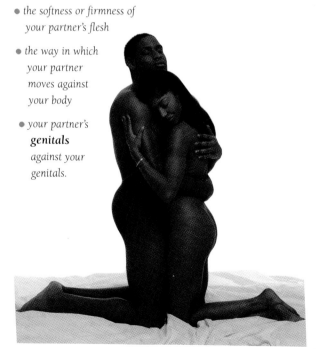

■ **Take time** *to savor the feel of your partner's naked skin against yours.*   25

Sharing the sex experience

It's the easiest thing in the world to assume that because you are having an amazing time during sex, your partner is, too. When you begin to feel emotionally connected, it's impossible not to believe that your experiences are shared, shiver for shiver. But in fact, this shared experience doesn't always happen.

When to let your hair down

If you can't assume that your partner feels just like you do, how on earth can you know when to really go to town? For clues as to when to make your move, try reading body language. Are her arms wide open? Is he actively pushing his body against yours? Or is her body language defensive? This includes crossing the arms, holding the body away from yours, or swerving the face sideways, so you kiss a cheek and not the lips. If you sense hesitation, take the hint and stop!

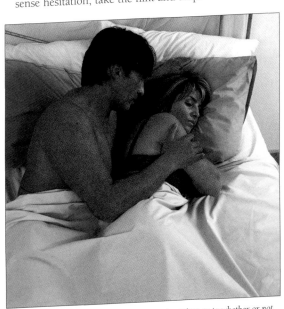

■ **Try to read the signals** *that your partner gives as to whether or not he or she is willing and in the mood for intimate contact.*

Simply communicate

When in doubt: talk; ask; open your mouth and let words come out. One reason why people hesitate to do this is because they are afraid of sounding silly. Or of somehow not pleasing this partner whom they want so much. But not communicating honestly is a big no-no.

It is always a mistake not to be yourself, or to let a partner think you are someone else. If you get trapped inside this other "you," the one who only wants to please, your partner never gets a chance to love the real you. Use the following "Yes/No" exercise, and talk truthfully.

THE "YES/NO" EXERCISE

This exercise helps you to clearly define your personal priorities. The rules are simple. In one week, say "yes" to three things that you really want to do, and say "no" to three things that you really don't want to do.

These things don't have to be sexual. It's the experience of saying a resounding "yes" or "no" that's important. You might decide, as one woman did, that you don't like your job, and so you resign. Or the next time the cashier at the supermarket gives you a hard time, you may decide to stand up for yourself and give it right back. The more you act, the more your confidence increases. And the more confident you feel, the easier it is to be yourself in bed.

KEY POINTS

- *Sex without eroticism can be fine. But sex with eroticism can be the best experience of your life.*
- *Eroticism is a work of art produced by two minds and two bodies.*
- *Eroticism can be anything from a suggestive remark in a crowded place to a bedroom decorated in a sexy theme.*
- *Never pressure a partner whose pace is slower than your own.*

What men expect

BOYS AND GIRLS are so alike as infants that it is suprising how many little differences creep in. Once they reach puberty they already have very different ideas about sex, and yet they actually experience very similar physical reactions when it comes to the great act. By virtue of possessing such different sexual apparatus, boys tend to discover sexual sensation earlier than girls, and this colors the rest of their sexual development.

What boys learn from their fathers

Traditionally, fathers have been distant or less involved in raising children than mothers. This leaves boys without many options for learning about sex – pornography or playground banter may be the only instruction available. So in purely technical terms, boys may not learn very much about sex from their fathers.

Boys are very likely to pick up a lot of their emotional attitudes from their fathers.

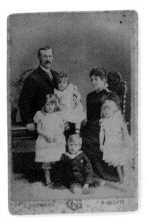

If a boy had an expressive father who was good at showing affection and talking about his emotions, then he probably got a head start. But if he had a father who was nearer the traditional model – remote and inexpressive – then, as a man, he may find it difficult to express emotion or display vulnerablity.

■ **Formal Victorian** *attitudes toward sex persist with some fathers today.*

Men who hide their emotions

A boy might well have learned from his dad that crying, kissing, hugging, getting upset, being scared, or showing any other loss of control made you a sissy, a wimp, or a mama's boy.

Psychologists say that you "internalize" the male role model that your father provides. One writer has called this internal model the "inner Arnie," as in Arnold Schwarzenegger.

The inner Arnie never lets down his guard and can never show any emotional or physical weakness. He represses strong emotions of every kind. Unfortunately, the inner Arnie can mean *hasta la vista* to a truly intimate, loving, and therefore satisfying, sex life.

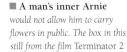

■ **A man's inner Arnie** *would not allow him to carry flowers in public. The box in this still from the film* Terminator 2 *contains a sinister secret!*

Sexual freedom for men

It's not all doom and gloom for boys. Being male has an upside: Boys are expected to be boys. In other words, they are tacitly encouraged to be sexually active and are allowed much greater sexual freedom.

Boys don't suffer from repressive "nice boy" messages. There can't be many boys who were told that "nice boys don't do it until they're married."

29

What boys learn from their own bodies

If there's one area where men have a head start on women, it's in the much underrated realm of **masturbation**. Since a boy's sexual organs are situated on the front of his body, they are simply impossible to ignore – with the result that the young owner becomes comfortable from an early age with the little quirks and sensitivities of his genitals. Boys get to know themselves in a way that most little girls don't.

Men and masturbation

No one would deny that masturbation is still a taboo subject. Your friends might cheer on tales of your latest conquest, but believe me, they don't want to hear about your five-fingered exploits. However, there's also no question that boys today are not subjected to the alarmist nonsense of yesteryear.

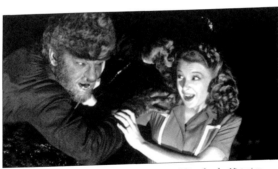

■ **Is this drooling,** *hairy-palmed, woman-grabbing fiend a Victorian perpetual masturbator or just a lycanthropic menace?*

 No one believes any longer that masturbation makes you go blind, gives you hairy palms, or transforms you into a drooling pervert.

In Victorian times, misguided educators identified masturbation as a source of moral degeneration. Among the contraptions devised to prevent masturbation was a metal jockstrap fitted with a sharpened spike.

Learning to "get off"

Believe it or not, all the masturbating that boys did, and probably still do, has positive implications for their sex lives. Because boys are more likely to enjoy lots of self-stimulation, they learn about their sexual responses early on.

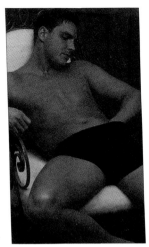

■ **Men learn** *a great deal about their sexual responses through masturbation, which is not considered nearly as taboo as masturbation for females.*

Chances are that by the time a boy loses his virginity he knows all about his penis and his orgasm, about what "gets him off" quickly, or about what simply turns him off altogether. It's only in recent years that women have begun to learn the equivalent information about their sexual responses before becoming sexually active.

Learning to slow down

But boys tend to fall short when it comes to slowing things down or taking a more rounded view of sex. For example, a man not be experienced at:

● *exploring non-genital* **erogenous zones**

● *bringing himself to the edge of orgasm, but not over it*

● *indulging in elaborate fantasies.*

Adolescent male masturbation tends to be penis-centered, with the emphasis on rushing to orgasm. Men need to overcome this if they want to become skilled lovers.

31

What boys learn from their male friends

Try as they might, parents are still not entirely comfortable with doling out comprehensive sex education to their children. And let's face it, kids aren't usually too comfortable when their parents try. So boys (and girls) are much more likely to learn about sex from their friends and fellow students.

Displaying sensitivity

Think back to your childhood and remember what it was like to be a young boy. Sensitivity and tact were probably not the order of the day. Boys tend to treat issues like sex in a fairly brutal manner. Male friends probably don't display much in the way of weakness or sensitivity – so other boys simply follow their example.

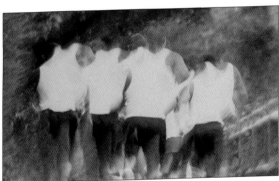

■ **Strength and endurance** *tend to come higher on the agenda than sensitivity when it comes to teaching boys how to be "real men."*

Talking about sex

On the other hand, some of these playground characteristics can be positive. Boys are able to talk about sex with a sense of humor that comes in handy later on. Among male friends, tales of sexual adventure don't have to be avoided or suppressed. And boys don't fall prey to the sexual catch-22 that girls suffer from – that she's a "slut" if she's sexually successful and "frigid" if she's not.

The softening of male attitudes

Men are inevitably being affected by the independence that women now take for granted. Women go out to work, achieve, earn money and promotions, and still take care of the home and the children if there are any. Many men are very supportive, but there are still a lot of guys who don't quite understand how the world has moved on.

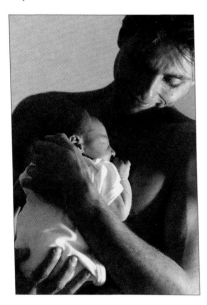

■ **The increasing** *number of "house husbands" is indicative of the many recent changes in male attitudes.*

Men in crisis

At work, women are demanding equal access and equal pay, and they are finally catching up with men. Women have also challenged traditional sex roles and gender limitations to reassess and reinvent their place in the world. By extension this means that men also have to change, but evidence says that not all of them are dealing with the prospect very well.

 Attitudes are shifting at home, too. Women expect men to help around the house, get involved in raising the kids, and be more considerate lovers.

Confusing messages about male behavior

Men get conflicting messages about how they are expected to behave. A glance through any woman's magazine tells you that women want men to perform several apparently contradictory roles.

> **Nowadays, men are expected to be sensitive, confident, gentle, bold, capable, sexy, fun, and serious by turns.**

New man, wild man

Having realized that the problem will not go away, men have made some efforts to redefine masculinity. First came the new man, who adopted "feminine" characteristics, such as sensitivity and nurturing, but threw out all the masculine ones. He wasn't very popular.

Recently there has been a backlash against "attacks" on traditional male values. Old-fashioned habits are in vogue: beer guzzling, skirt chasing, and dirty-joke telling. In the UK, this behaviour is seen in so-called "new lads." The trouble is they are very similar to the old lads.

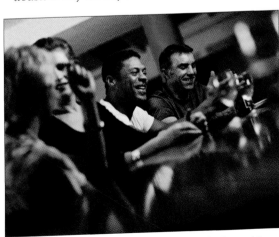

■ **It may be true** *that men have adopted more "female" characteristics, but drinking with the boys is still on the agenda.*

The complete man

Being a man in this day and age is obviously difficult. "Successful" masculinity involves many qualities, but luckily almost all of them can help men in the bedroom.

> *Assertiveness and sensitivity, a willingness to talk and to listen, and being emotionally empathetic are all qualities of a successful male.*

One writer has called this being a "complete man." If that sounds like too tall an order, men should think of it as being a man of parts. The first step in becoming this sort of man is to be prepared to talk, whether to their partner, to a therapist, or to other men. Since talking is a major component of wonderful sex, this can be excellent practice.

■ **You may consider yourself** *to be a complete man, but have you stopped to think what she wants?*

KEY POINTS

- *Boys learn from their fathers that sex is good, but they can also be taught to be so buttoned-up that they can't express their emotions.*
- *Boys learn about their own sexual responses early on, but tend to focus only on their genitals.*
- *From their friends, boys pick up unhelpful stereotypes about sex and relationships, but also become accustomed to talking about sex in a humorous and direct fashion.*
- *In the present day, being a man can be tricky; the challenge is to integrate greater sensitivity and openness with traditional male values.*

35

What women expect

UNLIKE BOYS, girls find out little about sex when young, and this can delay their understanding of sexuality. Sensuality may not be apparent until as late as the early 20s, although many female pop stars represent themselves in overtly sexual ways, which influences young girls. Some girls repress their sensuality until they feel they have reached an age when it is okay to be seen as sexual.

Growing up as a girl

If a girl had liberal, enlightened parents, they will probably have sat her down at an early age and told her about the birds and the bees. With luck, they will have found one of the excellent illustrated books on how babies are made. What they almost certainly won't have told her is anything about sexual pleasure.

UNSPOKEN MESSAGES ABOUT SEX

If parents feel uncomfortable talking about sex, the discomfort will show in their voices. Children or teenagers may wonder why they were cut you off when they asked questions, or why their parents awkwardly thrust a book on them. They will remember this reticence in later life, when it's time to think or talk about sex. Some parents say nothing at all about what to expect, which leaves girls with a very eerie impression of what sex is all about.

Secret lessons about sex

It's not just a girl's parents' early discussions that have an impact. It's also the examples they set. Mary said: "My parents actually thought it was sissy to kiss and hold hands. I now find it hard to know when to show affection." It can be difficult for girls with undemonstrative or protective parents to know when to show love themselves.

*Children unconsciously take in their parents'
attitudes about love and warmth. And when these
lessons are negative, there may be some
unlearning to do when they grow up.*

Girls: discovering sexual tension

As they grow older, girls may become aware of a tension
focused between the legs. They may touch the area with
their hands. They will not necessarily discover orgasm,
but the pressing and rubbing will feel good. Not all girls
discover their genitals, however, because they are
relatively tucked away inside the body, so they may never
fully discover sexual sensation during childhood.

*A girl's dreams may reveal that she is becoming
sexually responsive. For example, she may dream
of skiing, and experience a wonderful, sexual
feeling as she glides down the slopes.*

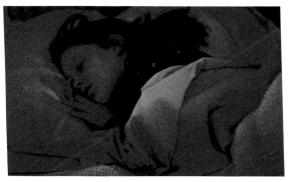

■ **Early indications** *of female sexual awakening can often enter the
subconscious in the form of dreams.*

Sexual changes take place in a girl's body for about two
years before she experiences her first period. During this
time she will grow breasts and pubic hair. She will also
still be growing in height. When her first period arrives,
her growth rate tails off. In general, the later she gets her
period, the taller she is likely to become.

Women who feel good about themselves

Women who feel good about themselves don't care if they don't get things right the first time – they know they can improve. They know they are capable of learning from their mistakes, and they don't get down on themselves.

Learn to be positive

Women who seek help with their sex problems often share something in common. They have been belittled, criticized, or "put down" by their parents.

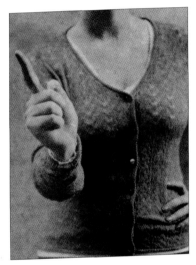

■ **If many of** *your childhood memories of your parents involve criticism of some type, you may be at risk of developing sexual problems later in life.*

 Criticism makes it hard for a growing child to develop confidence. Never put down your child – be constructive instead.

An inhibited or anxious mother provides no positive example from which to learn. Girls literally don't know how to be breezy and bouncy because there has never been anyone to show them. They probably need someone else from whom to learn more positive messages, and should seek out a role model or mentor to confide in, such as a favorite teacher, or the older sister of a friend.

The simple power of encouragement

Sometimes, in adulthood, people need encouragement to talk about sex. If a woman encourages her partner, she is likely to get the same treatment back.

- *Offer reassurance with words – "I love the way you stroke my breasts."*

- *Offer reassurance with gestures, such as strokes and hugs.*

- *Say "I love you" regularly – out loud.*

Asking for what you want

If you find it hard to ask for what you want, the "SHOULDS" exercise can help. Write down a list of ten actions you think you should take. These actions can but don't have to be sexual. Now number them in order of difficulty, and start with the least difficult action.

MAKING YOUR LIST OF SHOULDS

Your SHOULDS list may look like this: I should…

- *go out with my girlfriends more often*

- *ask the cute guy at work out for a friendly drink*

- *confront people who jump ahead of me in a line*

- *insist on more information when someone I work for doesn't give me enough*

- *walk away from my mother next time she criticizes me*

- *stand up to my father if he shouts at me*

- *visit my grandmother more often*

- *try out self-stimulation*

- *ask my doctor for contraceptives*

- *take unwanted presents back to the store.*

A hardening of female attitudes

Women are becoming more independent. Forecasts predict that one in six women will choose not to have babies or to live with a man. In contrast, 30 years ago, young women were expected to be wife, mistress, prostitute, housekeeper, and secretary – all essentially passive roles.

The mindset that went with being passive was that women expected to devote their time to everyone else's welfare but not on their own.

Women's passivity was reflected in their sex lives. They expected men to take the initiative. It was men who made the first date and knew what to do in bed. Women expected to be led and to be shown.

Changing expectations of gender roles

Then women changed. They insisted on more work that was better paid and that provided real opportunities to climb the career ladder. As they gained these things, women also gained confidence. Now they expected to be superwomen. They could do everything that men did and more. The catch was that they got exhausted.

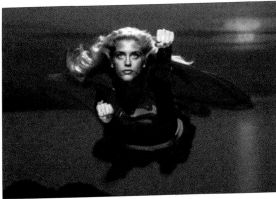

■ **Living up to the Superwoman ideal** *can be tough on today's working women. Juggling a career with a family and a relationship can leave a mere mortal feeling absolutely drained.*

Shared care in the home

Slowly women began to feel the unfairness of doing everything. If they were out there working at all hours, plus doing the housework, then why shouldn't men do the same? The problem was that men had become used to being waited on. They dug their heels in. And there wasn't too much women could do about it except weep over the dirty dishes. So then women grew angry. And anger affects sex. Men learned the hard way that they had to change.

Girls' expectations today

Nowadays girls expect boys to do housework. And boys are being raised to. Their support has improved loving relationships. But now both partners are tired at the end of the day. Men and women who want to have good sex find they have to make special time for it.

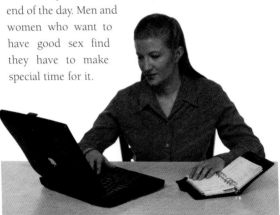

■ **Expectations** *among women have changed in recent decades. But even if there's work to do, it's still important to find time for relationships.*

KEY POINTS

- *Girls absorb unspoken messages about sex from parents. If these messages are negative, they need to work to overcome them.*
- *Women were once expected to be passive. Now they are equal with their partners.*
- *Women long for a good sex life but no longer believe this inevitably goes hand in hand with domesticity.*

First sex

MAKING LOVE FOR the first time is a sensitive occasion. Now, perhaps more than any other time, it helps to feel really in touch with your partner's desires and inhibitions. One rule of thumb is that if you feel something is not working quite as you would like it to, pull back and try again on another occasion.

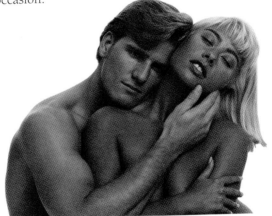

■ **Take the time** *to embrace after sex – it will give both partners a warm and precious feeling of being loved and wanted.*

Simple code of sex ethics

It's self-evident that the first time you have sex with someone your behavior is going to make a major impact. Your partner's senses will be on high alert, drinking in every impression you make. If this new partner is important to you, naturally you want to give the impression that you're a "nice guy". Here, the term "nice guy" applies to both men and women!

 "Nice guys" possess a code of honor where first sex is concerned.

The right stuff in bed

Nice guys do:

- *pay attention to a partner's verbal and body language*

- *take their time with sex*

- *use a great deal of touch and oral sex on their partner before going for intercourse*

- *use fingers during intercourse, on the grounds that both men and women adore getting extra stimulation*

- *stay awake, stroking and cuddling for at least 10 minutes after intercourse.*

Things to avoid in bed

Nice guys don't:

- *go for orgasm as fast as possible*

- *ignore a partner's needs*

- *get up and get dressed immediately after sex is finished*

- *judge the partner unfavorably after sex*

- *roll over and instantly go to sleep.*

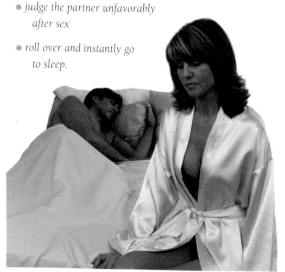

■ **Falling asleep** *immediately after sex can leave your partner feeling that you're only interested in one thing, and that can be very hurtful.*

Rescue tactics for first-time sex

First-time sex is rarely perfect, so
the following ideas may help:

- *be loving, affectionate, and
    full of caresses and kisses*

- *explore each other with
    hands and tongues*

- *talk about the not-so-
    spectacular first time,
    and reassure each other*

- *be patient. Understand that
    although some people can
    climax at the stroke of a
    finger, others may take
    time to relax.*

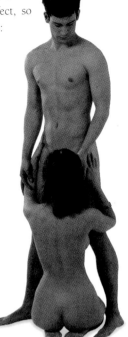

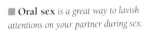■ **Oral sex** *is a great way to lavish
attentions on your partner during sex.*

 *If you want to have better sex, you will need to like
each other enough to persevere.*

Asking what your partner wants

Men and women can be reluctant to ask for what they
want in bed. The good news is that there are lots of other
ways of communicating sexually. One brilliant game to
play with your partner is the sexological exam. This is a
sex-therapy method that originated at the Institute for
Advanced Study of Human Sexuality in San Francisco.
Simply put, it is an adult version of "playing doctor."

 *The sexological exam helps you become more
comfortable with explicit touch, and encourages
you to talk about sex.*

The male sexological exam

Ask your partner to lie down naked on a bed in a warm, private room. Begin by finding out how his chest and nipples respond to touching and stroking. Gently stroke around his chest, then stroke or lightly press around the area of each nipple, using your fingertips. If his nipples become firm or erect, that shows they are sensitive to stimulation.

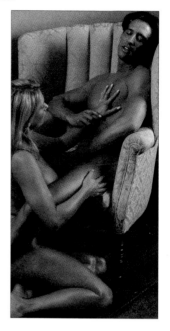

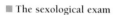
■ **The sexological exam**
will help you understand how your partner responds to touch. Begin by running your fingers over his chest.

Now transfer your attention to his pubic hair. Try tweaking and stroking it both lightly and roughly and see what effect this has.

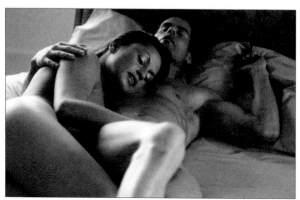

■ **Turn your attentions** *to his pubic area before you make direct contact with his genitals. Gently tease his pubic hair and watch his reaction.*

45

What to look for next during the examination

Your next port of call is your man's penis. Hold it in one hand and ask him to point out the areas that are most sensitive.

 Let him show you how he stimulates his penis, then give it a try yourself.

Don't bring your partner to orgasm. The aim of the sexological exam is to clarify for both of you which parts of his body are most sensitive.

Other noteworthy areas to explore...

Penis shape: The appearance of a man's penis is as individual as the appearance of his face. Ask him on which side he prefers to wear his penis when dressed, and ask if one side feels more sensitive than the other.

Foreskin: If he is uncircumcised, ask him to show you how far back he can comfortably move his foreskin. If he is circumcised, look carefully at the exposed penis where the foreskin would have been. Ask him what kind of sensation he feels here.

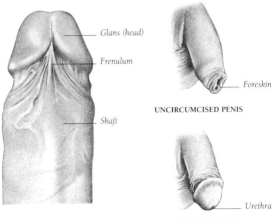

Glans (head)

Frenulum

Foreskin

UNCIRCUMCISED PENIS

Shaft

Urethra

STRUCTURE OF THE PENIS

CIRCUMCISED PENIS

Frenulum: On the underside of the penis, at the head, is a ridge of skin called the frenulum. Note if this is smooth, or if it is broken or scarred. Ask your partner what kind of sensation he experiences here.

Perineum: This is the area between the testicles and the anus. Gently run your fingers along the perineum and ask him how it feels.

Anus: Imagine his anus to be a clock and press gently but firmly at the hour positions around it. Ask him if any of these areas feel sensitive. If they do, remember them when stimulating your partner during later lovemaking.

Always wash your hands before and after examining or stimulating his anus.

Asking for what you want

It is essential when one of you does the sexological exam that the other partner also gets a turn. The more your partner explores your body, the more information you are able to give him about your sexual needs.

Don't forget, you must be naked for the sexological exam.

GIVING EACH OTHER VERBAL FEEDBACK

One of the rules of the sexological exam is that if you are the one carrying out the exam, you ask your partner for feedback with each new move you make. If you are the partner under examination, remember that the deal is that you voluntarily contribute information. If something feels great, tell your partner. If something has little sensation or feels uncomfortable, tell your partner about that, too. The whole point of this exercise is that it's a fact-finding mission, and those facts have to be communicated.

The female sexological exam

Men, begin by cradling your partner in your lap, having first made sure that you will be totally undisturbed. Begin with her breasts and nipples. In many ways the exam is similar to that for the male. But of course there are differences in the way each of you responds. Women's breasts, for example, often become much more visibly aroused than men's when stimulated.

Stroke or lightly press around her nipple area, noting any nipple erection or firming and swelling of the breast. Ask her to point out the most sensitive areas and to tell you how she prefers her breasts and nipples touched. See if there are any differences in response between the left and right sides.

Testing her genitals

Before you examine your partner's vagina and anus, lubricate your fingers with K-Y jelly (a greaseless and hygienic lubricant that can be bought in drugstores or supermarkets).

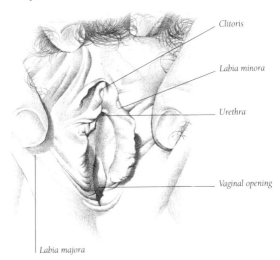

Clitoris

Labia minora

Urethra

Vaginal opening

Labia majora

STRUCTURE OF THE VULVA

Examine her genitals: First place your fingers on the outside of her labia, then at the opening of the vagina and just inside the vagina, and then on the base, the middle, and the top of the **pubococcygeal (PC) muscle**. (The pubococcygeal muscle is located on the floor of her vagina when she is lying on her back.) At each point along the muscle, ask her how much she would like it if your penis could hit that particular spot during intercourse.

Examine her anus: Imagine her anus to be a clock, with the 12 o'clock position as the point closest to the vagina. Press gently but firmly at the hour positions around it (on the outside), asking her which areas feel the most sensitive. The 10 o'clock and 2 o'clock positions are often the areas of greatest sexual sensitivity.

Examine her perineum: The perineum, between the anus and vagina, is rich in nerve endings and is always sensitive to stimulation.

Look in a mirror: Give your partner a mirror so that she can see her genitals. Point out to her the outer and inner **labia**, and then part them to reveal her **clitoris**, **urethra**, and the entrance to her vagina.

 Always wash your hands before and after examining or stimulating her anus.

KEY POINTS
- *First sex isn't always blissful.*
- *Patience and practice improve sex.*
- *How you behave affects how comfortable or uncomfortable your partner feels.*
- *The sexological exam is a great touch method for getting comfortable with each other.*

49

Journey to the interior

AS RECENTLY AS 50 years ago, human beings did not know what happened inside their bodies during orgasm. This was because sex had been such a taboo subject. Nice scientists did not undertake sexual research. So it took some exceptionally brave individuals to journey into those most secret regions.

The sexual world inside the human male

In general, men are more quickly and easily aroused than women, but after orgasm they usually have to wait much longer than women before they are ready and able to have intercourse again. The most obvious sign of male arousal is an erect penis, but this is only one of a number of physical changes.

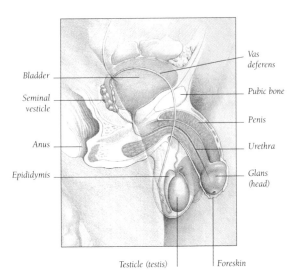

Bladder

Seminal
vesticle

Anus

Epididymis

Vas
deferens

Pubic bone

Penis

Urethra

Glans
(head)

Testicle (testis)   Foreskin

THE MALE SEX ORGANS

How sexual excitement works in men

Male sexual excitement works a bit like a two-way radio. When a man is turned on by physical stimulation, his skin sends sexy feelings to his brain. The brain promptly sends messages of encouragement to his penis, which responds by getting erect. Sometimes, it is the brain that gets sexy first – for example, when he has a sexual fantasy, or when he sees a beautiful woman undress.

 Amazingly, the penis can become erect within 10 to 30 seconds of stimulation.

Once sexual excitement really gets going, blood pressure rises, heart rate and skin temperature increase, pupils dilate, and, in some men, the nipples become erect. All of the body's muscles become spectacularly tense, breathing becomes almost hypertensive, and many men experience a visible sex flush.

How orgasm works in men

Physiologically, orgasm is a release of the muscular tension and engorged blood vessels that build up during sexual excitement. Subjectively, orgasm is a peak of physical pleasure.

Men recognize that orgasm is imminent when they reach the "point of no return" – a sense of inevitable ejaculation. At this point, the semen is pumped through the urethra by intense muscular contractions.

 The rhythmic muscular contractions of the penis during orgasm occur at exactly the same frequency as contractions of the vagina during orgasm.

Orgasm can lead to an altered state of consciousness. This, in most men and women, means simply a sense of being on a different wavelength, although not actually losing consciousness.

51

THE MALE'S SEXUAL HOTSPOTS

The penis is probably the male's most sensitive organ.
But just how sensitive it is depends on several factors,
including whether the penis is:

● *circumcised or uncircumcised*

● *curved or straight*

● *healthy or suffering from thrush, herpes, or genital warts.*

**The penis and scrotum naturally possess a
distinctive smell, which intensifies when a man is
aroused, and secretes pre-ejaculatory fluid.**

The male response cycle

The three stages of the sexual response cycle are desire,
arousal, and then orgasm. Desire is a hard-to-quantify
emotion, which some say is an attitude of mind and
others say is the product of hormonal activity. It often
blends with the next stage of sexual response, which is
arousal. Some men become aroused with little or no
physical stimulation, but others may need a great deal
before they are ready to progress to intercourse. As
stimulation continues by hand or during the thrusting of
intercourse, a man's arousal and excitement intensify,
leading to the final stage of orgasm and ejaculation.
Excitement then subsides as the man enters the
"refractory period," during which his body makes a
gradual return to normal.

Sexual response consists of three phases:

● *desire – you want it*

● *arousal – you need it*

● *orgasm – you've got it!*

The sexual world inside the human female

What goes on inside the female body during sex is surprisingly similar to what goes on inside her mate. Both sexes experience similar phases of sexual excitement, and both have similar types of orgasm. But there are a few differences – exciting ones. For example, very few men can have a second or third orgasm after the first one. But some women can.

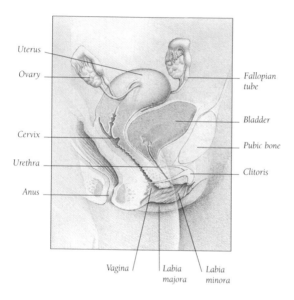

Uterus
Ovary
Fallopian tube
Bladder
Cervix
Pubic bone
Urethra
Clitoris
Anus
Vagina
Labia majora
Labia minora

THE FEMALE SEX ORGANS

How sexual excitement works in women

The first sign of female arousal is vaginal lubrication. The vagina lengthens and distends, and the vaginal walls become filled with blood. Women experience an erection of the labia and the clitoris. At the same time the breasts swell, the nipples become erect, and, on the inside, the uterus and the cervix begin to move upward. Heart rate and blood pressure increase.

53

How orgasm works for women

During extreme excitement, women reach a phase where the vagina does something called **tenting**. In effect, the vagina changes shape, resembling in cross-section a small, dome-shaped tent. During this phase, the walls of the vagina also exude a secretion.

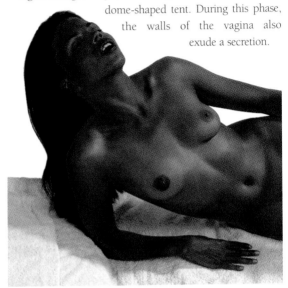

■ **During sexual excitement** *it is common for the face and chest to redden in a sexual flush, in both men and women.*

During sexual arousal, the genital area becomes so swollen that the clitoris seems to disappear. What actually happens is that the clitoris becomes hidden by the engorged genitals. These conditions, plus the sex flush, are the "jumping off point" for orgasm.

 Orgasm begins with muscular contractions as sexual tension is released. Women usually have 3 to 15 of these contractions.

Women experience a variety of bodily reactions to extreme sexual arousal, including jerking the limbs and body and even violent trembling. Sometimes the uterus and anus also contract during orgasm.

The woman's body after orgasm

Women differ from men in that the female body doesn't necessarily go back to "normal." Instead, it may return to the stage of extreme excitement experienced just before orgasm, and may climax several times.

The female's sexual hotspots

Women also differ from many men because they may derive extreme sensual pleasure from simple touch on sensitive parts of the skin. There are some women who become so aroused this way that they can climax from stroking alone.

For the majority of women the clitoris acts as the pleasure button.

In much the same way as the penis and the brain work together in the male, in women the clitoris functions as both transmitter and receiver with the brain. First it sends sexual signals to the brain, then the brain translates these signals into sexy feelings, and then the feelings are sent right back down to the clitoris and other parts of the body.

The female response cycle

A woman's sexual response cycle, like that of a man's, begins with desire. Arousal is the second stage, and while some women get aroused very rapidly and are ready for orgasm almost immediately, others take far longer.

In fact, some women need up to 45 minutes of stimulation before it is possible for them to achieve orgasm. During orgasm, the orgasmic contractions are very similar to those of a man. The majority of women then experience a loss of sexual and muscular tension as their bodies return to their normal physiological condition – the exception being the minority who go on to have multiple orgasms.

Orgasmic extras

No one orgasm is the same as another. Orgasms can be of different lengths and degrees of sensation. One person may have a climax they consider earth-shattering, while another person might rate a similar orgasm merely adequate.

The multiple male

Did you know that a very few men may experience multiple orgasms? American researchers William Hartman and Marilyn Fithian report that men have demonstrated this capacity in laboratory conditions. These men seem to have trained themselves to squeeze their pubococcygeal (PC) muscle so successfully that they effectively block off their ejaculate (semen) while still experiencing orgasm.

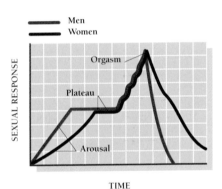

— Men
— Women

SEXUAL RESPONSE

Orgasm

Plateau

Arousal

TIME

■ **This diagram** shows and compares how a man and a woman might experience orgasm during a 30-minute sexual encounter.

The multiple female

It is likely that many more women are capable of experiencing multiple orgasm than actually do so; they simply don't receive from their lovers the kind of special stimulation needed.

To experience multiple orgasm, a woman needs unbroken stimulation and a very high degree of sexual arousal.

Some women experience multiple orgasms as gentle peaks of excitement that feel connected. Other women simply have one strong climax after another, each seeming to run into the next.

Multiple orgasm training

For him…

1. Practice flexing your PC muscle. Do this by trying to move your penis using only your internal muscles or by trying to lift a towel with your erect penis.

2. Gain testicle control. Either practice pulling your testicle muscles up toward your body – by regularly contracting your pelvic floor muscles – or fall back on the Beautrais Maneuver.

3. The Beautrais Maneuver is named after Pierre Beautrais, a New Zealand sex therapist. It consists of reaching around behind you when you are nearing "the point of no return," and pulling down firmly on your testicles. This inevitably prevents ejaculation.

4. Try to prolong an erection for as long as possible. Start by maintaining the erection for a minute each day for the first week, and then building up from there.

For her…

1. Increase your erotic arousal. Watch a sexy movie or develop your own sexual fantasies.

2. Delay your orgasm. Put it off, again and again, until you reach an extreme pitch of excitement. (Use a vibrator if you get tired.)

3. When you reach climax, continue with the stimulation.

4. Don't think that you are inadequate if, like many people, you are not able to climax more than once.

Safe sex and contraception

Safe sex generally means sticking to sexual practices where you protect yourself and your partner from sexually transmitted diseases (STDs) such as HIV.

 The best way to avoid STDs is to use a condom.

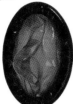 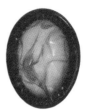 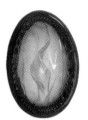

■ **Today's condoms** *come in such a variety of textures, shapes, sizes, and colors that there is one out there to suit everybody.*

Do's and don'ts of putting on a condom

Eighty-five per cent of men produce a few drops of seminal fluid at the end of their penis long before they ejaculate. This is why you should put on a condom as soon as there is an erection.

 Always squeeze the tip of a condom between thumb and forefinger as you put it on. An air bubble in the tip may cause splitting.

HIV and AIDS

HIV stands for human immunodeficiency virus. It is a virus that attacks the body's immune system. AIDS stands for acquired immunodeficiency syndrome. This is a condition caused by HIV that depresses the immune system and leaves you vulnerable to serious illnesses that would be fought off naturally under normal circumstances. You can catch HIV from infected people's bodily fluids.

 Never expose a condom to oil-based products, as they will weaken latex.

Levels of risk associated with sex

You are at an increased risk of contracting HIV from:

- anal intercourse
- intercourse without using a condom
- fellatio, especially to ejaculation.

You are at some risk of contracting HIV from:

- intercourse using a condom
- cunnilingus
- bites and scratches that break the skin
- mouth-to-mouth kissing if either of you has bleeding gums or cold sores
- sharing sex aids such as vibrators.

You won't get HIV from:

- dry kissing
- wet kissing, as long as neither partner has bleeding gums or cold sores
- stimulating the body with the hands
- stimulating the genitals by hand
- swallowing saliva, as long as neither partner has cuts in their mouth
- the bites of bloodsucking insects, sneezes, toilet seats, telephones, other people's beds or towels, swimming pools, shared food, or handshakes.

KEY POINTS

- **Men's and women's sexual reactions are very similar.**
- **Some women and a very few men are capable of multiple orgasms.**
- **Safe sex is vital to protect you and others from AIDS and other STDs. Make sure you use condoms properly.**

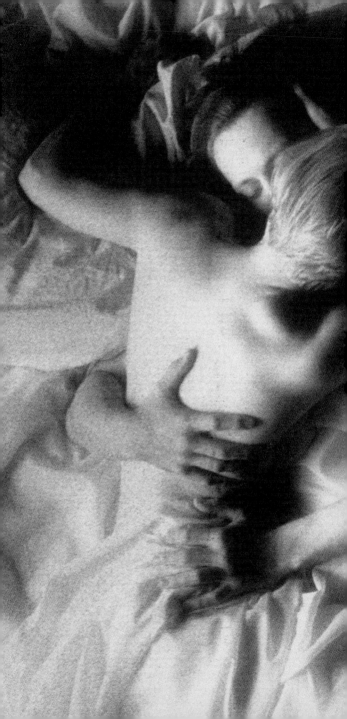

Part Two

Great Lovemaking

I believe that the best way to use sex manuals is to read them with interest, maybe get some ideas from looking at the pictures, but then to hurl the books into the corner of the room. Lover's tip: don't concentrate on perfecting a particular technique or position. Instead, enjoy your lover and every aspect of his or her personality. The real secret to good sex — along with being brilliant with the hands, tongue, and genitals — is to make your lover feel wonderful about him- or herself.

In this part...

■ Getting into position

■ Sensual massage

■ Love's variations

■ Gay sex

Getting into position

IN LOVEMAKING, PRACTICALLY anything goes – provided it's done with each other's consent and nobody gets hurt. Having said that, there are some ultrapopular sex positions that most of us use most of the time. That is probably because they are both pleasurable and offer intimacy.

The missionary position

The missionary position got its name (myth has it) from astounded natives, who spied on the love habits of Christian missionaries. I always feel that there's something humorous about the missionary position: perhaps it's the movement involved, or the actual face-to-face contact. Still, despite its comic potential, it's the sex position that allows for the most intimacy between two people.

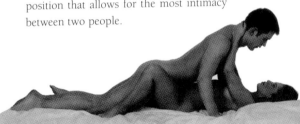

■ **The missionary position** *has the benefit of allowing eye contact between a couple, improving communication during sex.*

The missionary is the basic man-on-top position, in which the woman lies on her back with her legs apart, while the man penetrates from above.

Good points of the missionary position

The missionary position offers whole body contact – belly to belly, face to face. There is a maximum amount of skin contact and, because your faces are close, you can kiss and talk. And this position benefits from lots of variations.

Bad points of the missionary position

If the man on top is very heavy, it can be harmful. And if you want to avoid mouth-to-mouth contact – for any reason – this position makes that difficult.

If the woman is pregnant, the missionary position should be avoided after the sixth or seventh month of pregnancy.

Tips for perfect missionary sex

The man needs to take the weight of his body onto his forearms to avoid crushing his partner. Since he needs both hands to do this, it is helpful if the woman can reach down and guide his penis with her hand.

Varying the missionary sensation

Most variations on the basic missionary position involve the woman altering the position of her legs: drawing one or both of them up toward her chest, wrapping them loosely or tightly around her partner's waist, or putting one or both legs over his shoulders.

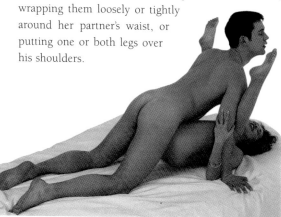

■ **For maximum penetration** *the woman can pull her knees close to her chest and rest her feet on the man's shoulders.*

Changes in a woman's leg position alter the tilt of her pelvis and the angle at which the penis enters, varying the sensation for both partners.

63

Woman-on-top

While the missionary position frequently misses the clitoris, the woman-on-top offers the possibility of a direct hit. And if you love being playful during sex, this position offers many possibilities. Woman-on-top is the reverse of the missionary. It is any position where the woman sits or lies astride the man.

Good points to the woman-on-top

When you are on top of your partner in a semi-kneeling position, it is easier to vary the angle of intercourse – for instance, by leaning forward so that your body is pressed against your lover's, or by sitting half or fully upright. And different angles mean different sensations.

In the woman-on-top position you can tease your man by slipping the head of his penis into your vagina and then pulling away again.

■ **When the woman** is on top of her partner, she is mobile and can take a more active role. This allows her to control the movements and sensations.

Bad points to the woman-on-top

It takes strength and fitness to maintain the thrust and pull of intercourse. If you are not in very good shape, the woman-on-top position can be hard work.

When sex educator Betty Dodson makes her female students practice a form of female thrusting, many of them rapidly collapse with exhaustion. And if your partner is much bigger than you are, it can be almost impossible for you to get both your knees on either side of him in order to thrust in the first place.

SIMPLE SEX EXERCISE

If you want to practice thrusting, get down onto your hands and knees, elbows on the ground, and thrust your pelvis forward and backwards. Keep the thrusting going for 3 minutes to 5 minutes if you are especially physically fit.

If you find the woman-on-top position tiring, sit upright and push off with your feet every time you rise from his penis.

Tips for perfect woman-on-top sex

If your man tends to come too soon, you can prolong your lovemaking by slowing your movements just as he gets to the brink and reaching down between you to give him a penile squeeze (see page 125). This squeeze involves firmly grasping the penis on the coronal ridge (the ridge around the head of the penis) between forefinger and thumb and squeezing firmly to prevent ejaculation.

If you adore kissing your man while thrusting, lie full-length along him and ask him to help you rise and fall by slightly lifting you as you thrust.

Varying the woman-on-top sensation

When you are on top of him, give him extra stimulation by brushing your nipples lightly across his chest. Vary your position by lying along your partner's body with both your legs outside his, or try sitting on top and facing away from him. If he wants to hold on to your waist or buttocks, he can use his strength to push you up and vary the depth of penetration.

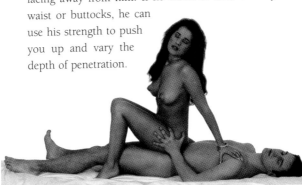

■ **Depth control:** *sit upright facing away from the man, then lean backward slightly. This allows the woman to alter the depth of penetration.*

While the woman is on top, you can alternate who takes control of the movements. While the man is lying on his back and his hands are free, he can control the tempo, but while his arms are supporting his weight, the man is left with little room to move at all.

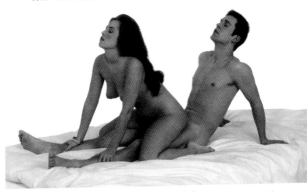

■ **Forward support:** *while sitting forward, the woman can support herself on her hands and use them to raise herself up and down.*

Sex from the rear

Rear-entry sex positions offer tempting and provocative alternatives to face-to-face sex. If your partner likes hand stimulation, it's easy to offer her this while thrusting from behind. If you enjoy playing games, this position provides powerful inspiration.

During sex from the rear, the man positions himself behind the woman, his penis against her buttocks, and inserts his penis into her vagina.

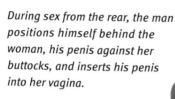

■ **The "doggy" position** *is a popular variety of rear-entry sex. While some women find it very arousing, others feel vulnerable in this posture.*

Rear entry can be done while lying down, kneeling, cuddling, standing, or sitting. And for those of you who believe rear-entry positions don't offer intimacy, you're wrong. Cuddling in the "spoons" position gives you sensual, whole-body contact during rear-entry sex.

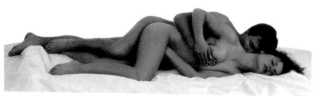

■ **The spoons position** *can feel particularly intimate, as the couple's bodies make close contact with one another.*

Good points of rear-entry sex

Rear-entry sex is erotic. It takes us back to primeval days when we copulated like other primates. It feels primitive, and where sex is concerned, that's hot. Men feel powerful as they thrust, and women feel seductively helpless as they open up their legs. And this position is versatile: you can do it standing up, bending over, or kneeling down.

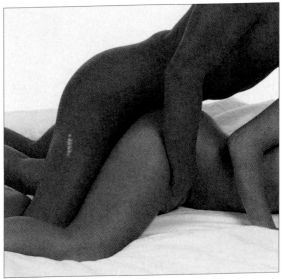

■ **Rear entry** *positions can give the man freedom to give his partner extra stimulation with his fingers.*

Rear-entry sex demands the least energy. For pregnant women especially, this has got to be the prime position.

Bad points of rear entry sex

If you are inhibited you might feel embarrassed in this position. And if you don't know your partner very well, rear-entry sex may feel unpleasantly impersonal. Finally, if you are in a relationship where there are a lot of power struggles, this position could be used as a method of domination.

Tips for perfect rear-entry sex

In the spoons position, since the couple are both lying on their sides, he can reach around with his top hand to stimulate her, or she can stimulate herself.

Varying the rear-entry sensation

The rear-entry position has more varieties than virtually any other sex position, from the intimate spoons to the more athletic wheelbarrow position shown below. Rear-entry sex also fits in well with the fantasy dominating-master/submissive-slave scenario.

If you enjoy playing sex games, rear-entry sex offers a great deal of variety.

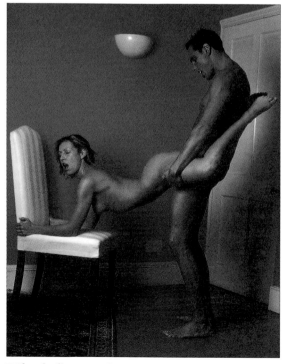

■ **The wheelbarrow:** *in this position the man lifts and supports the woman while she rests her forearms on a chair, wrapping her legs around his back.*

Standing sex

The *Kama Sutra* describes some terrific positions for standing sex. The "twining of the creeper" is a notable one. The man stands as strong as a tree trunk, and his fair partner (the creeper) wraps herself around him – arms, legs, and vagina clinging to every available surface.

In standing sex one partner, usually the woman, stands upright and leans back against a wall or other surface, while the man, also standing, penetrates her. Standing positions also include those where the woman leans forward and her partner takes her from behind.

Good points to standing sex

Most people associate this style of lovemaking with the inability to wait a moment longer. The great convenience of standing up for sex is that you can do it anywhere, so you don't have to waste time getting to the bedroom. Many people adore standing sex because it makes them feel daring, naughty, and passionate.

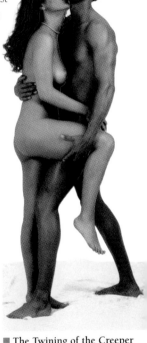

■ **The Twining of the Creeper** *is a sexual embrace defined by the* Kama Sutra, *which can be used to lead to standing sex.*

 Having sex while standing on two feet is pretty hard work, and it helps if you are a natural athlete, or if you have something to lean against.

Bad points to standing sex

If you are not athletic, standing sex is difficult to do since it is tiring. And if the man is much bigger than the woman, he must be strong enough to hold her up. If you are a woman who needs a lot of clitoral stimulation in order to climax, it is difficult with this position.

Tips for perfect standing sex

The classic love manual *The Perfumed Garden* recommends a standing position called "belly to belly." In this position the man inserts one of his legs between his woman's and, as he inserts his penis into her vagina, helps her lift one of her legs high so that her thigh is resting on his thigh. This way she feels opened up while he finds it easier to thrust.

Varying the standing sex sensation

One game described in the *Kama Sutra* uses the power of the imagination. The author Vatsyayana suggests that you make love in the style of different animals.

Most animal positions involve standing sex, where the woman leans over and the man thrusts from behind. In the "congress of a cow," for example, she leans forward with her hands on the ground while he holds her by the waist. He can then pull and push against her as he moves.

■ **Bending over:** *though pleasurable, this position can be very demanding for the woman and should not be adopted for any great length of time.*

71

Sitting sex

Sitting sex is fun. If you adore being playful in bed, this is a great sex position. And if your man really loves you bringing him off in an energetic and forceful manner, this is a good way to do it.

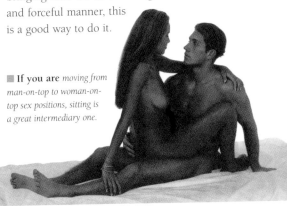

 ■ **If you are** *moving from man-on-top to woman-on-top sex positions, sitting is a great intermediary one.*

In sitting sex, the woman sits across her partner's lap, facing toward him or away from him.

Her legs are on either side of his, and either he thrusts from underneath or she lifts herself up and down on his erection. You can do this on a bed or on a chair. Both partners can sit upright, or the man can lie down while the woman sits on him.

Good points to sitting sex

The woman can get a regular rhythm going and pound down on him until he can't contain himself any longer. Women enjoy the sitting position because it allows them to feel in control and powerful.

Bad points to sitting sex

Sitting sex can be hard work for the woman. It takes energy and sound knee joints to keep thrusting. If the man dislikes being unable to move much, he might feel trapped and lose interest in the proceedings (although he can, of course, thrust upward from underneath).

Tips for perfect sitting sex

One of the most extraordinary sitting positions is that of the turning move. In this posture, the man lies on his back while his woman sits astride him and makes a slow, 360-degree turn on his penis – with the utmost care.

Varying the sitting sex sensation

There are several ways in which you can alter the sensation of sitting sex. For example, if you get tired from sitting up and thrusting, try leaning forward or even backward. Or, if you get hot about the idea of sex in the office, the sitting position fits well into a role-playing game of boss and secretary. And to vary the sitting sensation, try wriggling from side to side instead of up and down.

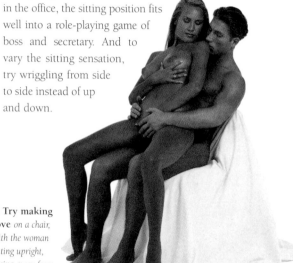

■ **Try making love** on a chair, with the woman sitting upright, facing away from the man.

KEY POINTS

- *The missionary position offers the most closeness and intimacy.*
- *The woman-on-top position enables the woman to control the depth of penetration and the pace of sex.*
- *Sex from the rear is a highly erotic alternative.*
- *Standing sex and sitting sex are done for fun or for passion; it helps if you're a bit of an athlete!*

Sensual massage

THE WAY WE TOUCH PEOPLE makes an impression from the moment we meet. If we touch with warmth and assurance, we invite warmth and appreciation in return. If we caress sensually, we provoke sensuality. With lovers, touch is the most immediate and important means of demonstrating love and providing reassurance. Good touch is a building block for good lovemaking.

Setting the scene for a massage

For a sensual massage to be truly successful, the surroundings in which it is given are as important as the technique and skill you bring to it. The room should be attractive, comfortable, carefully lit, and should provide adequate privacy.

Considering comfort during a massage

Make sure the room is warm and there are no drafts. Cold air makes the skin tense so that you experience touch as pain rather than pleasure. The best place to carry out a massage is on the floor because it provides a firm and steady platform. Cover it with fluffy towels, perhaps laid over a couple of flat rugs.

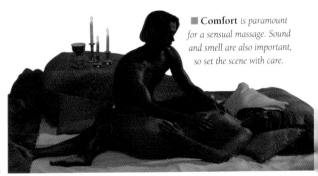

■ **Comfort** is paramount for a sensual massage. Sound and smell are also important, so set the scene with care.

Keep your fingernails short. Warm your hands by washing them in hot water, and take off jewelry that might come into contact with your partner.

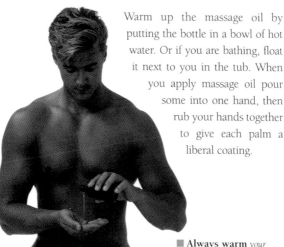

Warm up the massage oil by putting the bottle in a bowl of hot water. Or if you are bathing, float it next to you in the tub. When you apply massage oil pour some into one hand, then rub your hands together to give each palm a liberal coating.

■ **Always warm** *your hands and the massage oil before making contact with your partner.*

Aromatic delight for massage

The smell of incense or scented candles is an erotic addition to the sensual impression of the massage scene. The scent of the massage oil itself is also important – many herbalists and health stores stock oils suitable for massages. If you want a stronger smell, you can always add a perfume to these oils.

Massage oil should smell exotic. Baby oils and oils that smell like medicine or vegetables are not sexy.

Aural pleasure for massage

Some people like soft and tasteful music playing in the background during a massage session. But choose carefully: loud music or heavy rock is not suitable for massage; both detract from the sensual atmosphere.

Ten golden rules for an amazing massage

A massage doesn't have to be with a committed partner to feel good, but it does feel sensational to offer your light finger strokes to the one you love. It isn't about slapping the palm of your hand on your partner's naked skin, but takes preparation and consideration. If you and your partner want to have the most fantastic massage experience, you need to follow a few rules:

- *respect your partner's requests*

- *honor any agreement you make in advance of the session, for example, that intercourse is not on the agenda*

- *keep your massage movements slow*

- *be aware of the sensations you receive when giving a massage*

- *try to tune into your partner's reaction to a massage gift*

- *never foist a massage on someone who says they don't want it*

- *make a point of gently asking your partner for feedback*

- *when it's your turn to be massaged, remember to give your partner plenty of tactful feedback*

- *ensure that you have privacy*

- *make sure that the room, your hands, and the massage oil are warm.*

Sensational circling massage strokes

Although there are several classic massage strokes, one such stroke – circling – is the foundation for all others. If you can get the hang of circling, you can use it on every part of the body.

Performing the circling stroke

Place both hands, palms down, on the shoulders (it's best to start with a back massage), and move them firmly in opposing circles. Work your hands out and away from the spine, progressing slowly down along the back and over the buttocks. Then work back up to the shoulders. Repeat twice.

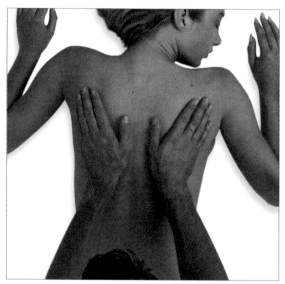

■ **For the circling stroke** *it is important to synchronize your hands in smooth, fluid movements.*

Varying the pressure of your strokes

Varying the pressure of your stroke is the secret of turning a routine massage into a sensual experience. A strong massage feels thorough and "medical"; a lighter massage is pleasurable and sensual; a fingertip massage is arousing and erotic. Begin with a firm touch to prepare the skin for arousal and gradually progress to a fingertip massage.

 Never massage directly on the spine or on any other bones – this hurts! And remember to ask your partner for feedback.

The most sexual massages

There are some very specific forms of intimate massage that can bring incredible pleasure, but they should only be performed after the rest of the body has had touch attention first. Preparing the skin for touch will make the final genital massage feel even more erotic. Before you move down to those most personal areas, make sure you pamper the back, the front, the arms, and the legs.

Genital massage for her pleasure

The three genital massages below can be performed on their own or in a sequence – you choose the order.

 During genital massage, always be sure that your fingers are slippery with oil.

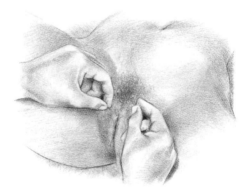

① The gentle hair torture
The idea here, of course, is not to torture, but to elicit an exquisite, pricking sensation that travels straight from the pubic area to that delicate sex organ, the clitoris. Using both hands at a time, pull her pubic hair gently and in small tufts. Work your way slowly – tuft by tuft – from the top of her pubic hair and travel gradually down each side of the labia.

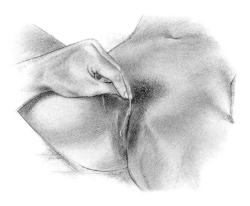

2 The duck's bill

Shape the fingers of one hand into a "duck's bill" and hold them above her clitoris. Pour warmed massage oil over the fingers so that the oil slowly seeps through and runs down onto her genitals.

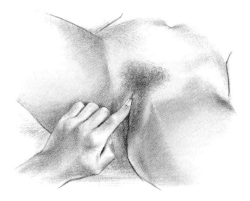

3 The clitoral maneuver

Using a well-lubricated finger, circle the head of the clitoris at a steady pace, then change direction. Keep the pace even. After 20 circles each way, rub the tip of your finger lightly up and down the side of the clitoris – 20 times on each side. Now rub backward and forward just below the clitoris 20 times. Finally, rub down from the clitoris to the vagina, and then back again, 20 times.

79

Genital massage for his pleasure

When giving your man genital massage, remember that your aim is not to bring him to orgasm. If orgasm happens, it's a bonus. If it doesn't happen, you will still have given him wonderful sensations. Begin by pouring a little warm oil into your hands and liberally applying this to your man's genitals.

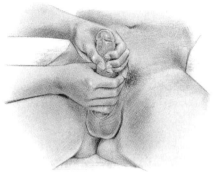

① The corkscrew
Rub the shaft of his penis between the palms of your hands, twirling it as you would a stick if you were trying to start a camp fire. In a variation of the corkscrew, you twist your hands in opposite directions—at the same time—around his penis.

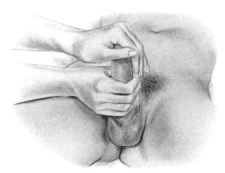

② The lemon squeezer
Rub the head of his penis with your cupped hand while holding the penis with your other hand. It helps if you close your eyes and actually feel your hand brushing across the surface. Circle the head of his penis very gently, first moving your hand ten times clockwise, and then ten times counterclockwise. Use steady strokes.

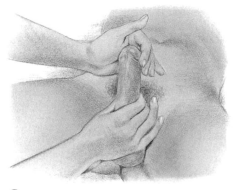

3 Hand over hand

This is like the game in which you repeatedly bring your hand from underneath a pile of other hands and place it on top, never breaking the rhythm. In this intimate version, however, you slide your cupped hand over the head of the shaft of the penis. Before it gets to the base, bring your other hand to the penis head and repeat the downward stroke, so that the shaft is never without a hand sliding down it.

Don't be afraid to hold his penis firmly – it can take a lot of pressure. If you are in doubt, ask him to place his hand over yours and squeeze himself.

KEY POINTS

- *Massage is a great method of learning sensuality.*
- *If you stick to simple guidelines it's hard to go wrong, because massage feels so nurturing.*
- *When giving a massage, experience it as a sensual event yourself.*
- *To create the most sensuous atmosphere for good touch it's wise to set the scene first.*
- *The basic stroke is a "circling" stroke. Even if you never use another one, this will always feel great.*
- *An intimate genital massage is a gorgeous way to finish an erotic touch session.*

81

Love's variations

HAVING SEX IS NOT only confined to intercourse. Sex is one of the great human drives and, as such, it can be enjoyed in a relationship with yourself. Or when penetration is not the order of the day, hands and mouths can provide exquisite pleasure. Alternatively, you may enjoy role-playing during sex and thrive on activities such as bondage.

Self-love

Self-love teaches you about your personal sexual response. Once you know this, you have established a solid footing for a good sexual relationship. Self-stimulation also helps build up self-confidence. This may sound surprising, but masturbation makes you feel desirable.

Self-stimulation

Most men discover masturbation as boys because their sexual organs are positioned on the outside of the body and are therefore easy to discover. More women than men come to masturbation later in life, since their pleasure button – the clitoris – is hidden inside their labia. Men gain more sexual knowledge and more sexual confidence at an earlier age than women.

■ **The external placement** *of the male sex organs means that the man is able to develop an understanding of how they work at an early age.*

Learning about sexual reponse

When it comes to learning about sexual response, some women do not catch up with men until they are in their 20s or even their 30s. These women may expect men to teach them about sexual response, and this can be tough on men, as there is no reason why a man should know more about a woman than she herself does.

Know your own love patterns

New York sex therapist and educator Betty Dodson holds classes for women that include the experience of masturbation. The women masturbate themselves (not each other) within a group. What becomes fascinatingly clear is that each woman approaches self-stimulation differently. She touches different parts of her body, moves in special ways, builds up to climax uniquely, and experiences orgasm in a number of different ways.

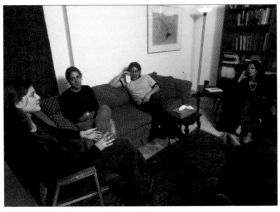

■ **A forum for discussion** *on masturbation can be particularly helpful in assisting women to overcome inhibitions about their bodies.*

This is why it's so tough for men to know how a woman gets turned on. There could be a dozen different ways. Intercourse works best when both partners are thoroughly familiar with their sexual response and can bring that information to each other.

83

Discover your sexual response pattern

If, by some chance, you don't yet know your masturbation pattern, here is a safe routine of exploration. Naturally this needs to be done in privacy. Spend an hour or so getting comfortable with yourself and your body, and follow these guidelines.

1 *You might start with a warm bath and run your soapy hands all over your skin, feeling the sensation as they glide and caress.*

2 *Next move to your bedroom and, using oil or talc, massage your body.*

3 *Move your hands to the genitals last.*

4 *When you reach the genitals, simply massage them as you have done the rest of the body. Note any really good feelings this self-massage brings and begin to build on them, focusing on the spots that feel special.*

On a second occasion follow the same formula, but spend less time on the whole body and more time on the genitals. Continue to build on the stimulation you give to the really sensitive areas. You are not actually aiming at orgasm – just exploring your sensations. If orgasm happens that's okay, but it's not the end goal.

Using a vibrator

Most people do end up discovering climax using the method just described. You may find that your body wants to move about or that you feel like calling out when you get really excited. Have no fear about doing any of these things. They are part of your response. However, if the sensations feel good, but climax still proves elusive, then it's a good idea to try using a vibrator.

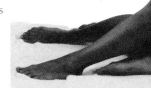

Mutual masturbation

Another great value of masturbation is that it can be used to enhance sexual intercourse. The majority of women find it hard to climax from intercourse alone. But over 80 percent of women can climax from self-stimulation. This tells us that including fingers during intercourse is a sensible idea if you want to climax.

Hands on for masturbation

Mutual masturbation lies at the heart of sex therapy methods. The theory is that masturbation is an important stage of sexual development and that if, for some reason, you miss out on self-stimulation, you miss out on an important building block.

When his fingers are needed for stimulation

Women need finger stimulation:

- *when they want sex to be focused solely on them*

- *as a preliminary to intercourse*

- *as an accompaniment to intercourse when it is otherwise difficult to climax (including when the sexual position, such as sex from the rear, doesn't give enough stimulation)*

- *as an alternative to intercourse when pregnant.*

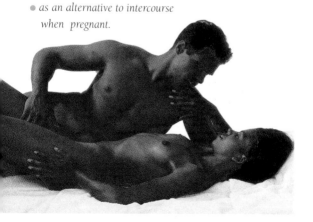

When her fingers are needed for stimulation

Men need finger stimulation:

- *when they want sex focused entirely on them*

- *as a preliminary to intercourse*

- *when they are older and the penis possesses less feeling*

- *when they just prefer an extra turn-on*

- *when they find it hard to climax without it.*

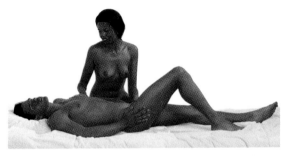

USING HER FINGERS FOR SEX FOCUSED ENTIRELY ON THE MAN

Masturbation myths

Contrary to Victorian propaganda, masturbation will not cause blindness, deafness, flu, insanity, or death. The notion that each teaspoonful of lost semen weakens you by the equivalent of a lost pint of blood is also totally without foundation.

Masturbation is a harmless and natural expression of sexuality. It is not addictive to the exclusion of all other forms of sex.

Human beings can enjoy many different forms of sexual expression. The only people who are truly addicted to masturbation – that is, they can't leave themselves alone, day or night – are seriously disturbed men and women. They are suffering from a form of mental illness and for them compulsive masturbation is only one of many symptoms.

Oral sex

Oral sex is the second great alternative to penetrative sex (the first being stimulation by hand). It is subtle, strong, sensitive, and varied. It feels amazing, provided you can overcome inhibition, and it offers truly exquisite pleasure.

The recent popularity of oral sex

Strange as this may sound to people who have grown up since the 1970s, oral sex was barely practiced, let alone discussed, before then. Of course this is an exaggeration, but huge numbers of men and women lived their lives without ever discovering it. If anyone did get to hear about it, it was seen as an aberration or a sexual deviance. Nice women didn't do it. Proper men wouldn't entertain the notion.

The "sexual revolution" of the 1960s and 70s changed all this. The breakthrough came when *Cosmopolitan*, the women's magazine, published an article on cunnilingus by Al Goldstein, which *Forum*, the sex magazine, wouldn't touch.

What is fellatio?

Fellatio consists of manipulation of the penis by mouth. You might start by treating the penis as an ice cream cone, holding it at the base with one hand and licking it all over, running your tongue up and down the shaft. Then, when it is covered in your saliva, take the penis between your lips and slide your mouth gradually down it to the base, then back again.

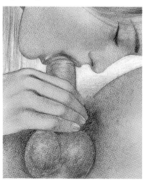

■ **Take his penis** *in your hand, place it between your lips, and move it around in your mouth with your tongue.*

87

Performing fellatio

To perform fellatio, move your mouth up and down the shaft, or you might experiment with sucking. Or you can try fellating the head only, including hand stimulation at the same time. It is up to you to decide if it's okay for your partner to climax in your mouth. If it isn't, you can substitute your hand or a tissue.

If we are talking large penis and small mouth, try to cover your teeth with your mouth; otherwise your lover might experience a nasty nip.

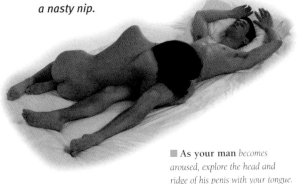

■ **As your man** *becomes aroused, explore the head and ridge of his penis with your tongue.*

What is cunnilingus?

Cunnilingus consists of manipulation of the clitoris by tongue. For really sensational cunnilingus, your head needs to be right between her thighs and preferably slightly below them so that you can stroke your tongue upward against her clitoral shaft. From here you can occasionally insert your tongue into her vagina.

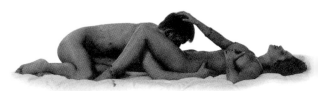

■ **The secret to good** *cunnilingus is not to pursue one stroke for too long, unless your partner has specifically requested that you do.*

Performing cunnilingus

Experiment with the tip of the tongue, and then the blade of the tongue. Try stimulating one side of the clitoris, and then the other, always from underneath. Ask her for feedback, so that you learn what she likes best.

 Some people enjoy sucking the clitoris, but don't suck the clitoris too hard, or you will bruise it and make her numb rather than aroused.

Simply sensational oral variations for him and her

For an extra-special oral treat, try the following:

● the "butterfly flick" consists of flicking your tongue lightly across and along the ridge on the underside of the penis. Another special mouth stroke focuses the movement of your whole mouth only on the coronal ridge (the ridge around the head of the penis) – an area of great sensitivity

● the "tongue twirler" consists of featherlight tongue twirling on top of the clitoris itself. Another version is to swirl the tongue in circles on the head of the clitoris, and a third version is to flick the tongue from side to side immediately underneath the clitoris.

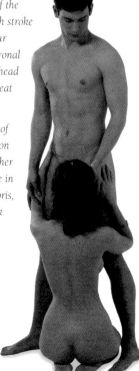

■ **Once you have** mastered fellatio you may be able to perform it without the aid of your hands, leaving them free to caress your partner's body.

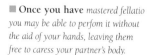

A little light bondage

Among the sex games that adults play is the controversial one of domination and submission. Most individuals have no interest in seriously pursuing this sexual variation but many ordinary men and women do enjoy the milder aspects of playful restraint.

When bondage is acceptable

Silk ropes and scarves flimsily tied, the warmth of mild spanking, the sting of a light cane—all of these are ingredients of on-the-edge sexual activity. Many men and women, when pressed, will admit to a fantasy of being held down by a lover and made to feel absolutely helpless.

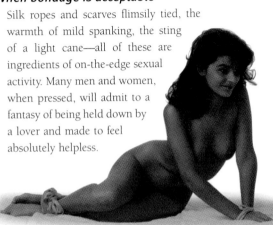

■ **For a gentle introduction** *to bondage games, try using silk scarves or ribbons as shackles – and maybe as blindfolds, too!*

Laying down the boundaries of bondage

It is vital that before you let loose with your imagination you have a very clear idea of what is going to be acceptable to your lover and what isn't. If you don't know, you need to find out well in advance.

One couple who developed an interest in bondage drew up some clear guidelines between them to ensure the game never crossed the bounday of what each found acceptable. If either shouted "Stop!" or "No!" or "I can't take it any longer" each agreed to take no notice. But if the partner being dominated spoke an agreed code word, all activities were to stop immediately.

Never put yourself into somebody else's power if you don't trust them or if you don't know them.

Playing bondage games

You might experiment with bondage by:

- *giving your partner boundaries to his behavior and punishing him if he moves beyond them. One punishment might be light caning or spanking. The game is more fun if the boundaries that you choose are impossible to stick to*

- *tying your partner to the bed with silk scarves and tickling and teasing her to climax*

- *blindfolding your partner after you have tied him by one wrist to a piece of furniture, then announcing that he must obey you completely. Sex toys, such as vibrators and dildos – anything safe – can come into their own here.*

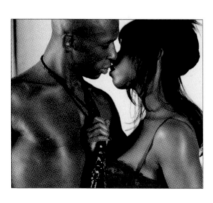

■ **Remember:** *as long as the two of you agree to your particular sex act, respect your agreed boundaries, and no other party is involved, you are hurting no one.*

KEY POINTS

- *There are many variations of sex, such as mutual masturbation and oral sex, that are perfectly acceptable when they are done in privacy between consenting adults.*
- *Self-stimulation is an excellent way of learning about your sexual responses.*
- *A little light bondage is great fun provided you trust each other completely.*

Gay sex

HOMOSEXUALS HAVE FOUGHT prejudice for years, and they are still doing so in certain corners of the Earth. However, gay people manage to live happily in many major cities. San Francisco, for example, has long been known as a gathering point for gay men and women. Cities are considered by many to be an escape route from rural areas where a gay lifestyle is still not seen as acceptable. London, for example, accommodates over half of all the homosexuals in England.

Homosexuality

Years of experience as a sex therapist have shown me that gay sex problems tend to be along the same lines as straight ones. The solutions to impotence or premature ejaculation are similar regardless of your gender preference. However, the social and emotional atmosphere accompanying the choice of a gay lifestyle is not. In this chapter I therefore tackle some of the emotional issues such as telling your parents about your sexuality.

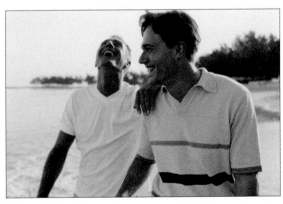

■ **Gay relationships** *are in many ways parallel to heterosexual ones; the problems and pleasures of being emotionally attached to someone are similar.*

What does it mean to be a gay man?

Some gay men choose to live a virtually identical life to their heterosexual counterparts as far as work, recreation, bonding, and families are concerned. Other gay men opt to live differently, spending time bar-hopping, enjoying constant casual sex, dressing in recognized "gay" styles, and mixing mainly with other gay people.

How do you know you are gay?

Many gay men say they knew from an early age that they were not the same as other boys. Even if they didn't know this, or felt confused, puberty – and with it the dawning of sexuality – often made their feelings clear.

 It may take some young men until their early or mid-20s to feel certain that they are gay.

Telling your parents you're a gay man

Many people advise breaking the news that you are gay in a very personal way. But instead of saying bluntly, "I am gay," it may be gentler to say, "I've fallen in love with a friend who happens to be a man." Most counselors recommend that you think carefully before telling your parents about your sexuality.

If one parent is likely to be hostile, start with the sympathetic one. For all the disowning parents, there are many with positive reactions. One 75-year-old woman said, "What does it matter? He's still my son."

What can you expect from your parents?

Even if your parents are broad-minded and loving, they will experience some shock. They will need to come to terms with many of the same things you did, such as the fact that you may never become a parent.

 Be patient with your parents and be prepared to talk things over, possibly many times.

93

Lesbianism

A lesbian is a woman who loves women and, in most cases, expresses that love through sexuality. She feels emotionally attached to women, rather than to men, and is more likely to live with a woman. A lesbian is like any other woman, except she prefers women as partners.

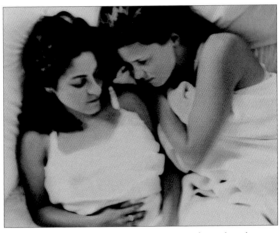

■ **Many women** *realize they are lesbians at an early age, but others may have several male partners before deciding on a preference for women.*

Finding out you are gay

Many lesbian women do not know they are gay until they reach their 20s. Many try, unsuccessfully, to enjoy heterosexual relationships first. In fact, there is a large number of women with children from former heterosexual relationships, who reach their late 20s before they comprehend that they are lesbians.

Lesbian lifestyles

Lesbians do not live particularly differently from heterosexuals. Recent figures show that two-thirds of lesbian women have always had the same sexual partner. Many lesbian households include children, either from previous heterosexual partners or through artificial insemination.

Telling your parents you're a lesbian

The process of telling one's parents about one's sexuality is much the same for lesbians as it is for gay men. Some parents are unhappy and rejecting. Again, if you fear you might be shut out of your parents' lives, don't tell them about your sexual orientation. On the other hand, you may be pleasantly surprised by your parents' reaction. One positive mother, when told by her 22-year-old daughter that she was a lesbian, said, "As a matter of fact, there have been times when I thought I was, too," and was supportive ever afterward.

Women who are confused about their sexuality

Some women feel confused about their sexuality and may become lesbians only after a period of bisexuality. Other women have absolutely no doubt about their feelings from early childhood on. They know that they love women, and, thanks to more information available now about gay options, these women suffer little confusion about their sexuality – although they have to deal with prejudice.

It is common for gay individuals brought up in the countryside to migrate to towns as soon as possible, because it is much easier to pursue a gay lifestyle in a larger community.

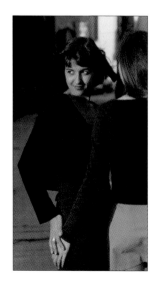

■ **Public displays** *of affection between lesbians may be easier in a cosmopolitan town, as attitudes are probably more relaxed than in a small, rural community.*

95

Bisexuality

Many people believe that bisexuals have the best of both worlds, that, when it come to sexual partners, they literally have twice as many choices as either homosexuals. But bisexuality doesn't quite work like that.

What is a bisexual?

A bisexual is a man or a woman who is able to relate sexually to both men and women. Many male bisexuals remain married to one woman but have extramarital relationships with gay men. Many female bisexuals have serial relationships, which may be with either men or women. Of course there are also men and women who go in for equal sharing of their sexuality with both male and female partners.

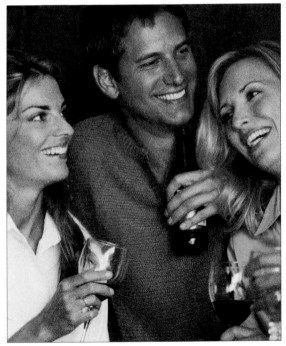

■ **Many people** *are attracted to both sexes, although it is estimated that only 10 percent engage in sexual activity with both men and women.*

A Freudian analyst might say that bisexual women have a deep-seated need to reexperience closeness to a mother figure.

Bisexual dilemmas

Some heterosexuals and homosexuals are wary of bisexuals and criticize them for their "flexi-sexuality." Their attitude stems from the belief that bisexuals are really gay people who refuse to be up-front about their sexual orientation and who disguise it under the label of bisexuality. This doesn't take into account those men and women who are truly "fifty-fifty" in their sexual preferences and who relate equally well to both sexes.

Telling others you're bisexual

Since bisexuals often spend their early years trying to understand their sexual behavior, they are often unable to tell anyone much about it. It can be confusing to be attracted to both sexes, but exciting, too. If you want to tell your parents, only reveal intimate details if you feel certain your parents can cope with them.

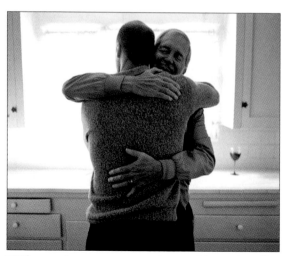

■ **When coming out** *to your parents, be prepared for an unfavorable reaction, although you might be pleasantly surprised.*

97

The facts about gay sex

There are a lot of myths about homosexual behavior, focusing mainly on the large number of partners gay men are supposed to have and the types of sexual activities they prefer. A major British survey in 1994 came up with some interesting and unexpected findings.

Gay for life?

The statistics showed that although many people reported same-sex experiences at some time or other during their lives, very few people reported same-sex activities during the year immediately previous to the survey interviews.

The study made it quite clear that many men and women experiment with gay sex but, after doing so, revert to a heterosexual or celibate lifestyle. Of course, there is a core group of people who are fully gay – but this seems to be a much smaller group than was previously estimated.

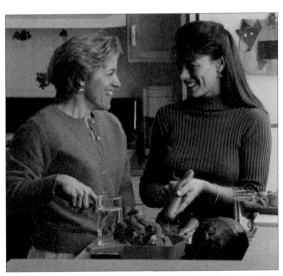

■ **Gay experiences** *may well be a transitional phase for some people, but for many others, being a lesbian or a gay man means making a commitment to a partner that may well last a lifetime.*

For gay men, first-time sex happens mainly in their teens and twenties. Among lesbian women, first-time sex could happen at any time during their lives.

Getting the most out of gay sex

There is not much difference between gays and heterosexuals when it comes to sex problems. Impotence or inability to climax are the same whatever your gender preference. The same therapies and medications are available, with the same results. There are differences in emotional anxieties, however, since the fact of being gay in a world mainly oriented toward heterosexuals can be difficult. There are many excellent specialized counseling centers – usually located in cities – that can help. Look up gay hotlines in a telephone directory, or buy a copy of a gay magazine or newspaper and check the counseling ads.

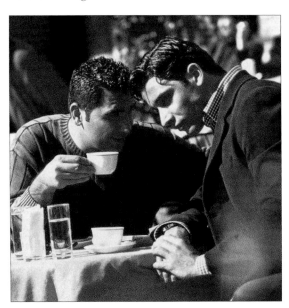

■ **Gay newspapers and magazines** *may help you make contacts and meet a partner if you experience difficulty in finding gay people to talk to.*

99

Gay issues

The major issue for gay men and women is, of course, acceptance by the community they live in. But there are also other specific issues encountered on the path to acceptance.

Parenting when gay

There is often criticism of the fact that some gay men and women bring up families. Yet research about the children of lesbian mothers, carried out in Britain during the 1980s, showed that the offspring were as well balanced as anyone else.

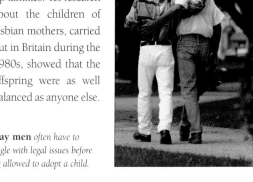

■ **Gay men** *often have to wrangle with legal issues before being allowed to adopt a child.*

Research on homosexual fathers indicates that they may well make better fathers than many heterosexual ones. They may be more empathic and able to help children work through problems constructively.

Equal rights for gays

The outbreak of AIDS in the early 1980s reversed a lot of the gains that gay men and women had achieved. Gay parenting continues to be condemned by the religious right, even though it is becoming legally and socially more acceptable. In many countries, however, the age of consent for gay men is higher than that for heterosexual men.

If you are interested in combating prejudice, you will find names and contact numbers for campaigning groups in the local gay press.

Making gay friends

If you live in a city, you will have little difficulty finding places where you can make friends. But if you are in a backwater, life can be horribly lonely. You may be able to find like-minded friends through the help of chat groups on the Internet, or the classified ads in the paper.

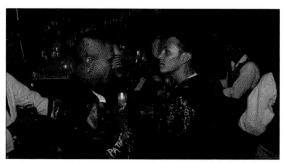

■ **The clubbing scene** *in cities makes meeting other gay people easier.*

Dealing with homophobia

The only way to eradicate prejudice is through education and personal contact. This will happen when:

- *more perfectly respectable men and women let it be known that they are gay*

- *more school children are informed about heterosexuals and homosexuals as a matter of course*

- *more institutions, such as the police, teaching professions, and armed forces, accept homosexuality.*

KEY POINTS

- **Gay men tend to become sexually active mainly in their teens and late twenties.**
- **Gay women tend to discover their lesbianism later, perhaps after heterosexual relationships.**
- **It's important to combat prejudice, especially when homosexual dads appear to be better at parenting than many heterosexual fathers.**

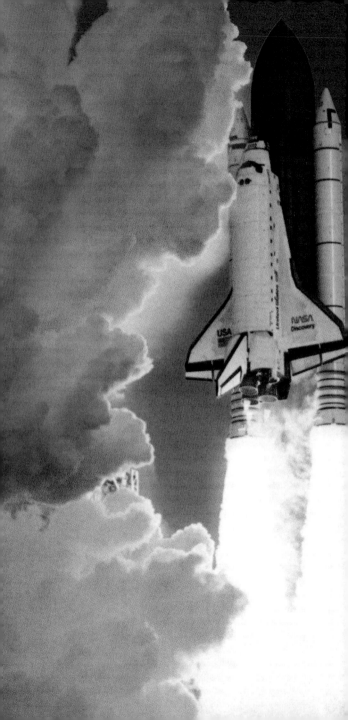

Part Three

The Further Reaches of Sex

We grow up believing that everyone else is like us. It's quite a learning experience to discover that we are not all the same. Many of the most ordinary-seeming people regularly enjoy a sex life that is extraordinary by our own standards. After years of writing about sex, I've come to understand that even if we don't engage in the many unusual sex practices that apparently fascinate others, we still want to hear about them. It's as if we need to work through them in our heads to know if these idea are for us or not. In Part Three we look at sexual lifestyles, sexual religion, and the fun accessories of sex.

In this part...

■ Sex for explorers

■ Extra-special interests

■ Troubleshooting

■ Sexual dilemmas

Sex for explorers

SOME PEOPLE SEE SEX as a journey of adventure. Searchers into the far reaches of sex believe that they will find new facets of themselves emerging from the intensity of their experiences. Or they may simply need a more ritualized sexual routine in order to feel aroused. Whatever the ultimate aim, these people believe that sex needs to be enhanced and extended.

Sexual accessories

There is a sizable minority of people who like making elaborate preparations for sex. They enjoy contemplating the event in advance, getting ready for it and planning how to surprise their lover. These are the men and women for whom corsets, stockings, bath oil, and ice cubes offer a particularly sensual slant to the sex act.

Erotic role-playing

Do you have a burning desire to play nurses and doctors? A plain white coat will do for the doctor. Some underwear specialists offer a rather fetching genital strap with a red cross embroidered on the front. A nurse's uniform can also be purchased from a specialty retailer.

Perhaps you are content with playing the virgin bride. Lace-topped stockings, lacy white underwear, a flimsy see-through negligee, and a scattering of red rose petals are easy to obtain.

EROTIC LACE UNDERWEAR

Playing the dominatrix

Maybe your mood is darker. Shiny black tight-fitting bustiers, fishnet stockings, long black boots, a satin sleep mask, and a black military cap could offer a more daring atmosphere for your lovemaking.

Bathing for sensual excitement

Bathing is an exciting preliminary to sex. There is something about the slippery sensation of shiny, soapy skin next to soapy skin that gets the senses racing. Peppermint massage oil offers the skin quite an extraordinary sensation – as does the impact of a mouth made cold with ice cubes or hot with tea or coffee. Try using hot and cold in rapid succession during oral sex.

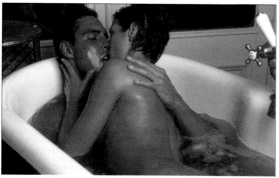

■ **Experiment in the bath:** *the feel of your partner's wet, slippery skin against your body is an exciting prelude to sex.*

 Be careful about using "stimulatory" creams offered by sex-aid advertisers. Most don't work.

The simple smells of sex

We are all far more affected by our sense of smell than we realize. How a partner smells is crucial to how attractive we ultimately find him or her. This includes genital smells, which can be a prime **aphrodisiac**. Certain musks are supposed to have stimulatory effect, and there are scents and perfumes devised around musky ingredients. 105

Sex aids and toys

The list of possible sex toys is so long that many people need to find a toy box for all their belongings and then keep the goodies under lock and key. Sex toys are as old as the hills, and until the discovery of electricity, there were very few new ones. Simple toys like silken ropes for tying up and blindfolding your partner, and peacock feathers for teasing them are centuries old and still popular today. But now, thanks to our harnessing the power of the elements, we can choose from any number of variations of the latest sexual invention – the vibrator.

PEACOCK
FEATHER

Greek and Roman sex toys

The ancient Greeks used stone dildos to deflower high-born virgins, although with the passing of time the canny temple priests substituted themselves instead. The Romans made dildos of leather or of fig wood, and sex toys were unashamed features of the houses of ill-repute.

Sex toys during the Renaissance and beyond

During the Renaissance dildos were made of glass, and the customers for these objects were often nuns. The infamous Catherine de'Medici (1519–89) once found four such dildos in the trunk belonging to one of her ladies.

With the advent of rubber, clitoral stimulators were manufactured. A French mail-order company offered women a rubber sheath that fitted over the fingers, with soft points at the tip. They also advertised double-ringed stimulators to be fitted over the penis.

Sex toys for men and women

The vibrator is said to be the first truly original sex toy to be invented since the dildo. (Of course, prior to the invention of plastic and the discovery of electricity, they would have been impossible to manufacture.) Electric massagers have been around since the late 19th century, and vibrators became popular during the mid-1960s.

Men's sex toys

From vibrating penis rings that massage the male member to anal plugs that stimulate the **prostate gland**, toys for men can provide sensational variety.

- *Pulsating penis sheaths enclose and manipulate the penis.*

- *Penis rings fit around the base of the penis and help maintain an erection.*

- *Vibrating penis rings fit around the base of the penis and offer extra sensation.*

- *Anal plugs and anal vibrators stimulate the prostate gland.*

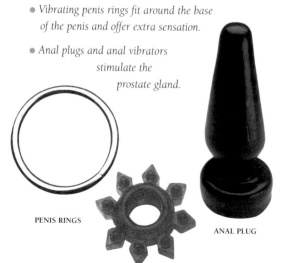

PENIS RINGS

ANAL PLUG

Women's sex toys

Many women are only just beginning to feel comfortable with the idea of sex toys.

- *Small "ben wa" balls that fit inside the vagina; some versions vibrate*

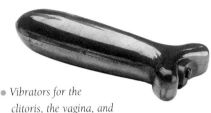

- *Vibrators for the clitoris, the vagina, and the anus, as well as vibrators for the G-spot*

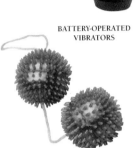

BATTERY-OPERATED VIBRATORS

- *Harnesses and dildos for women who want to play at being men*

- *Vibrating eggs for vaginal stimulation*

BEN WA BALLS

Oral sex toys

Try the following for added flavor in your sex life:

- *strawberry gel*
- *chocolate-flavored condoms*
- *chocolate body paint.*

Tactile sex toys

Try using the following tactile toys to make sex extra sensual:

- *feather duster*
- *soft leather paddle*
- *giant feathers*

108   - *fur and fabric massage gloves that include a vibrating egg.*

S&M toys

Toys for S&M lend themselves well to role-playing:

- *soft wrist restraints*
- *soft, long-stranded whips*
- *riding whips*
- *PVC thongs*
- *rubber-shining fluid that gives a spectacular gleam to rubber clothes*
- *collars and leashes*
- *removable tattoos*
- *fake handcuffs.*

■ **Try wearing** *a collar to play the sex slave, and satisfy your partner's every need while he or she leads the way.*

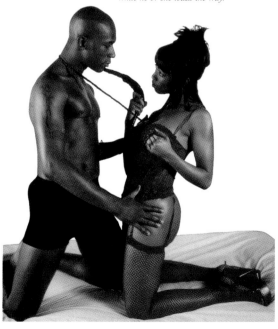

The ultracool condom

Condoms not only protect us from pregnancy and sexually transmitted diseases such as HIV, they can also be considered sex toys if you use them with imagination.

 Condoms are tested for safety to within an inch of their life. Great weights are hung from them and gallons of water are suspended in them.

The latest condom designs

Condoms got a new lease of life with the discovery of rubber (previously they were fashioned out of materials such as animal gut). Today they are available in the thinnest layers of latex. They are ultraflexible and are usually lubricated so that they don't cause unpleasant friction during intercourse.

Nice girls do carry condoms

For years men have been used to equipping themselves with condoms in advance. Women haven't. They have had to learn that it's not only okay to carry a supply of condoms in their purse – it's insane not to.

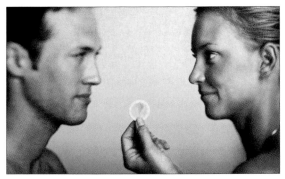

■ **Gone are the days** *when carrying a condom was the man's responsibility.*

 The message that women should carry condoms has meant throwing out the belief that "nice girls" don't plan their sex lives in advance.

Advanced sex positions

For those who want to experiment, here are some wonderfully old-fashioned names and sex positions – straight out of the 17th century.

The Lyons stagecoach

This is a woman-on-top position where he sits up, but leans back on his arms, while she sits astride him – also leaning back – with her feet planted square on the ground.

The Horse of Hector

In this woman-on-top position, the man lies on his back with his knees up and his feet square on the ground. She sits up during penetration, her knees on either side of him, and leans back against his thighs for support.

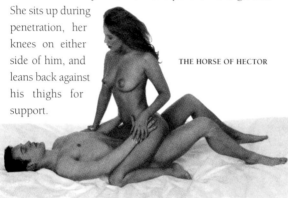

THE HORSE OF HECTOR

Cuissade

In this rear-entry position, she lies on her back with her legs hooked over his hips and he enters her "from behind." This gives the sensation of rear-entry, with the advantage of being able to kiss and caress each other, making this a tender rear-entry alternative.

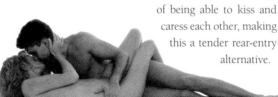

CUISSADE

111

Anal sex

Although anal sex is commonly associated with gay men, many heterosexual men and women enjoy it too. The anal area is rich in nerve endings, and activities such as rimming, and anal intercourse can be very exciting.

Provided you are scrupulously clean and do not go directly on to vaginal intercourse afterward, anal sex is hygienically safe.

How to have anal sex

To try rimming, moisten both your fingertip and your partner's anus with a suitable lubricant, such as K-Y jelly. As your partner becomes more relaxed, insert the tip of your finger half an inch (2 to 3 cm) into the anus and finger the inside edge in circles. Some women are profoundly turned on by simultaneous anal rimming and the clitoral stimulation.

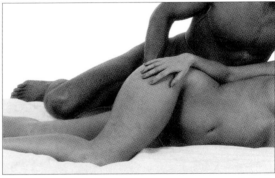

■ **Anal stimulation,** *if performed in the appropriate way, can be highly arousing for both you and your partner.*

Warning: anal sex between consenting adults is not legal in some countries.

Think of your partner's anus as a clock face: the 12 o'clock position is nearest the vagina or testicles. The most sensitive points are probably at 10 o'clock and 2 o'clock.

Relaxing is the key to anal sex

The keys to anal penetration without pain are: one, for the man to pause as he penetrates so that the woman consciously relaxes her back passage; and two, to use a lot of lubricant. Take anal penetration slowly and try to relax the anal sphincter muscles as much as possible.

Men possess sensitive anal nerve endings, and may love their partner to finger-massage them and to stimulate the prostate gland, which lies at the back of the upper wall of the anus.

What if your partner objects to anal sex?

Never do anything to anyone against their will. If your partner objects to anal sex, accept that it isn't going to happen. Still, a partner with uncertain feelings may agree to go ahead slowly, and with the guarantee that you will stop on request.

If, after going some way, something happens to make your partner want to stop, agree to go back a stage. This doesn't mean that the activity is put on total hold, but that your partner gets the opportunity to talk about whatever is making him or her nervous.

KEY POINTS

- *Specialized sex requires certain exotic pieces of equipment, such as lingerie, costumes, restraints, and sex toys.*
- *Although the condom is a contraceptive it can also be used as a sex toy.*
- *There are several unusual sex positions that many men and women like to experiment with.*
- *Anal sex, although still illegal in some countries, is regarded as very enjoyable by many couples.*

Extra-special interests

NOBODY KNOWS WHY some people develop erotic desires for unusual objects or obscure parts of the body. But the reality is that a few men and women (mainly men), through no conscious choice, are turned on, for example, by a rubber boot or a plastic raincoat. Possibly at some impressionable time in childhood a connection is made between unconscious sexual arousal and that object.

Sexual fetishes

Fetishes change with the times. The objects of people's passions 200 years ago would simply not excite us at all today. For example, Chinese men thought that a tiny foot, the result of the appalling and crippling cruelty of binding women's feet, was the sexiest item imaginable. Victorians thought that ankles were erotic. We don't find these same things as exciting today. So what are the fetishes of the 21st century and what determines their content?

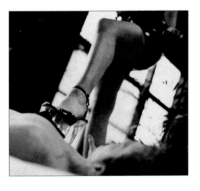

■ **Shoes and feet** *were the object of sexual fascination hundreds of years ago, and are still among the favorite domain of fetishists today.*

Who gets fetishes?

Many of us probably have minor fetishes, such as a special attraction to breasts or slim buttocks, but this doesn't prevent most of us from enjoying a regular sex life.

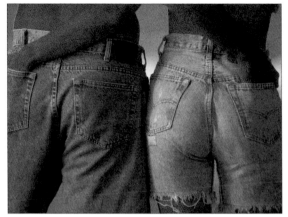

■ **Many people** *have mild fetishes for perfectly harmless and common triggers for arousal, such as the sight of a well-shaped rear in demin jeans.*

 If you have a major sexual fetish, it will almost certainly influence your relationships.

It is mainly, although not always, men who are fetishists. The current theory as to why men are more affected focuses on the fact that men are more responsive to what they see than women are. Because of this predisposition, men are more likely to pick up and focus on some eye-catching object.

How do we get fetishes?

We learn to be fetishists much as we learn anything else. A boy sees an object and then, probably accidentally, experiences sexual sensations. Next time he gets to be feeling sexy, the memory of that object comes into his head. And so the object and the eroticism are paired. If the boy masturbates during this learning period, the idea becomes even more embedded in his brain. For example, if a guy remembers getting erections while being changed on a rubber mat by his mother, he can get stuck on that association. Forever after, rubber means feeling sexy. Well, that's the theory anyway!

115

Five of the best fetishes

There are several common fetishes that are generally considered to be pretty kinky. Here are five of the best.

The Cinderella complex

Sufferers from the "Cinderella complex" are into shoes. Many men adore women wearing incredibly high heels because of the masochistic connotations; they want those heels to walk all over them.

Golden showers

Some couples adore urinating on each other. Many couples do this in the shower or in the bath.

Hair fetishism

Some men with "trichophilia" (the technical term for a hair fetish) actually snip off strangers' hair, creeping up behind them in the street or on public transportation.

Mud wrestling

It's quite common for men to fetishize the sight of two naked women rolling round in a sea of mud. The sexual excitement arises from seeing nude people getting filthy.

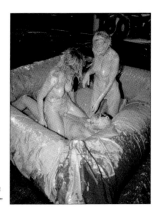

■ **Cavorting** *naked in a pool of mud can be a profound turn-on for those who enjoy getting "dirty."*

Rubber ware

Rubber fetishists are into PVC or rubber boots, raincoats, and aprons. Many wear latex underwear, and some even sleep on rubber sheets. Costumes, such as nuns' habits, skirts, and hoods are also part of the specialist clothing that is available.

The turn-on of transvestism

Transvestites are people who become sexually excited by cross-dressing – that is, by wearing the clothes of the opposite sex. Contrary to what many people believe, the majority of male transvestites are heterosexuals. Although they like dressing in female clothing, most of them still want sex with female partners. Most transvestites are men, and because they get aroused from the very femininity of women's clothes, they tend to indulge in extreme female fashions, such as high heels, frilly lingerie, and brilliant red fingernails.

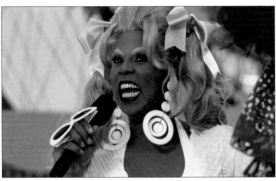

■ **Transvestites such as** *American celebrity RuPaul tend to be outlandish in their extreme liking for traditionally feminine accessories.*

What is a transsexual?

A transsexual is someone who has gender dysphoria and feels that he or she is actually a member of the opposite sex. Both males and females can be transsexuals and will probably have realized from an early age that they are different. In adulthood, it is possible to "reassign" a person's gender through hormone treatment and surgery.

Changing gender

In some countries, to qualify for sex-change surgery, you must prove you can live openly as a member of the opposite sex for 3 years. During this time, male or female hormones may be prescribed to help with the transition.

117

Male-to-female surgery

Male-to-female surgery consists of castration – amputation of the penis and testicles. The skin of the scrotum is retained and used to line the inside of an artificially created vagina. These male-to-females do not have a clitoris, but many of them report that the pubic mound, the area just above the new vagina, becomes highly eroticized. Electrolysis is used to remove unwanted body and facial hair. Estrogen stimulates the breasts to grow, which some transsexuals then choose to have enhanced with cosmetic surgery.

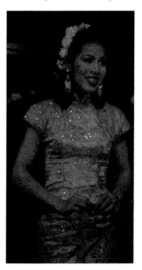

■ **Thailand** *is renowned for its "ladyboys," transsexuals who have had or are planning sex-change surgery.*

Female-to-male surgery

The masculinization process is started by prescribing androgens (male hormones), which encourage beard growth, general muscular change, enlargement of the clitoris, and sometimes baldness. The surgery includes a mastectomy; then a scrotum is constructed from the labia, and synthetic testes are inserted to resemble male testicles. Constructive surgery for a penis has not been very successful, and many transsexuals prefer to retain the enlarged clitoris – which sometimes grows to as much as 3½ inches (9 cm) as a result of the androgens.

For every female-to-male operation performed, there are four male-to-female operations.

Dangerous sex – what not to do

It goes without saying that any sex where violence, mutilation, and torture are involved is highly dangerous. Steer clear of the sexual practices described below.

Unprotected sexual intercourse and AIDS

If you don't know that your partner has a clean bill of health, practice safe sex (see page 58).

Autoasphyxiation

Some people deprive themselves of oxygen during sex in the belief that it will enhance orgasm. One method of autoasphyxiation is to hang yourself just to the point of unconsciousness. Another is to cover your head with plastic. Both can – and often do – prove fatal.

Cutting edges

Anything that involves cutting is potentially dangerous. Open wounds carry the risk of HIV infection.

Foreign objects

Some people pursue the curious hobby of stuffing unusual objects into orifices such as the vagina or rectum.

 Sharp objects in the vagina can perforate the uterus and cause a serious infection.

KEY POINTS

- *Fetishes range from bizarre (intercourse with rubber boots) to dangerous (autoasphyxiation).*
- *Most fetishists are men.*
- *Transvestites are mainly heterosexual men who get sexual satisfaction from cross-dressing.*
- *Transsexuals may be confused about their gender identity. Some seek gender-reassignment surgery.*
- *Some sex fetishes and practices are dangerous and should always be avoided.*

Troubleshooting

SEX PROBLEMS CAN happen to anyone. Maybe a lover's cruelty has damaged your emotional responses or perhaps your difficulty has arrived out of the blue. Your first move should be to talk things over with your partner. This will help you to feel less alone. And when you decide you want to find a solution, it always helps if your partner works with you. But there are, of course, other options for you as a single individual.

The three most common sex problems

The odds are that everyone will experience a sex problem at some time in their life.

It is normal to experience the occasional sexual failure.

Sex is one of those activities that cannot be controlled by will. Instead, it is controlled by something called the autonomic nervous system. Put simply, this means that sometimes your mind takes over even when you don't want it to. If your mind decides it is upset or angry, it may overrule your desire to make love. This can be pretty annoying. How you deal with these off moments affects how you experience sex the next time you have a go at it.

Fortunately for those with sex problems, there are many methods of solving them.

The most common sex problems you are likely to experience are impotence or premature ejaculation, if you are male, or inability to experience orgasm, if you are female. Just as there are a number of causes for these upsetting disruptions, there are also a number of solutions.

1. Impotence

Men may get just one bout of this or it can be a recurring problem. Impotence may have a psychological origin, such as stress, depression, guilt, or anxiety. A man may react badly to a particular partner simply because he doesn't find them attractive or even because he dislikes them. Or the causes may be physical. Diabetes, circulatory diseases, alcohol-related disorders, hormonal disorders, and certain medications – most notably antidepressants, antihypertensives, and diuretics for high blood pressure – can all interfere with sexual response. Even heavy smoking has been implicated.

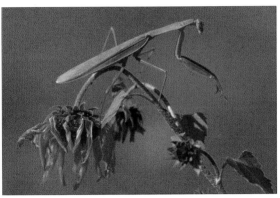

■ **If the male** *praying mantis knew his partner was going to eat him alive, he might well suffer the ultimate performance anxiety!*

2. Premature ejaculation

Premature ejaculation is considered mainly a young man's problem. It tends to be associated with anxiety, inexperience, and having sex under conditions where the participants are anxious to end the sex act quickly.

Fortunately, premature ejaculation is one of the easier sex difficulties to improve. There is a simple, do-it-yourself training routine that is covered later in this chapter, which helps in most cases. However, a tiny percentage of men need drug therapy to solve the problem.

121

3. Inability to experience orgasm

Some women are unable to climax through intercourse or, less commonly, through masturbation. They may not yet have discovered what works for them, they may suffer from inhibition, or perhaps they don't get enough stimulation during sex. In these cases, masturbation can help a woman learn to climax. Occasionally, some women may lack an adequate supply of testosterone, a hormone which is responsible for sexual desire and arousal.

The Hite Report found that only 30 percent of women climax during intercourse (compared with 82 percent during masturbation).

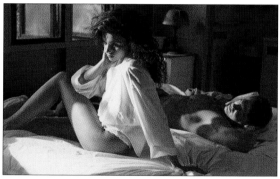

■ **If she is unable** *to reach orgasm, it may be that she needs more – or a different sort of – stimulation than she's been getting.*

Less common sex difficulties

Retarded ejaculation is a difficulty in climaxing for men. The man may grow excited, and he may want to climax, but ejaculation doesn't happen. It usually responds to sex-therapy methods, or occasionally testosterone.

Women's problems include vaginismus, when the vagina goes into spasm. This causes pain and can make penetration impossible. Vaginismus may be assisted by tranquilizers, which encourage overall relaxation of muscular tension, or by simple exercises.

Do-it-yourself sex therapy

There are a number of sex-therapy exercises that you can do at home. It makes sense, however, before embarking on these, to see your doctor so that physical problems can be ruled out.

Touch, touch, and more touch

Sensate focus exercises are the basis of do-it-yourself sex therapy. They consist of touch and massage exercises done by a couple so that each partner learns what does and does not feel sensual.

Sensate focusing exercises must be done for several weeks. In the first sessions you agree not to have intercourse. Then you learn how to massage each other, excluding the genitals (at least for the first couple of weeks). The purpose is to learn about your response to touch, and to give each other good sensual feelings.

 Remember: in sensate focus exercises you are trying to give pleasure rather than orgasm.

Getting him going again

Once a woman has learned the sensate-focus massage, her partner is likely to be experiencing an erection, partly because of the sensuality of her touch and partly because all pressure to "perform" is removed.

The next step is to climb on top of him and very slowly lower yourself onto his penis. You then stay there, hardly moving at all – just enough to keep his erection up.

If he loses the erection, all you have to do is climb off again and reapply the massage technique until he regains his erection. As he gets used to the feeling of you enclosing him, his confidence will grow and the erection will last longer. Once he can sustain an erection, you can build up to normal intercourse.

123

Finding her first orgasm

When you have both enjoyed the basic sensate focusing exercises, the man sits, usually propping himself up against something, and the woman sits between his legs and leans back against him. He needs to be able to reach around her so that his hands have access to her genitals. It is his task to explore her sensual reactions. Once again, the couple's aim is not to achieve orgasm. They are simply discovering what sensations she feels – then building on them.

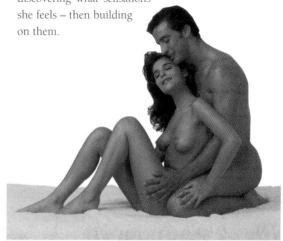

■ **When attempting** *to find her first orgasm, a woman should be sure to always tell her partner what feels good, as well as what she doesn't like.*

Adding to her climax

Once the woman has either achieved climax or has got to a point she feels unable to pass, the couple is encouraged to add a vibrator to the proceedings. A vibrator offers stronger stimulation than fingers. Sitting in this posture is warm and reassuring. The woman can easily guide her lover's hands if she wants to so that he learns through her where to touch and what kind of pressure to give.

If the orgasm-finding exercise works well, the woman may have a climax. But she may reach a certain point, then find it hard to go further.

124

Using the penile squeeze

The penile squeeze is an exercise for men with premature ejaculation. When he says he is going to come, you grasp his penis and press just below the glans. Release when he says that the urge has gone and then massage his penis until his erection comes back. As he gets used to this, his confidence will grow and he will trust he can sustain an erection without ejaculating.

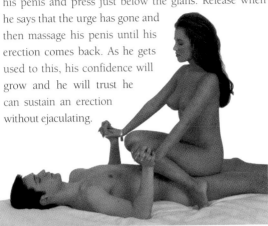

■ **When attempting** *to overcome his premature ejaculation, interrupt your gentle thrusting only to apply the squeeze technique.*

This exercise is also designed to make sex last longer. The woman sits astride her partner and thrusts gently while he remains immobile on his back – until he can last for 15 minutes. He signals when he thinks he is reaching the point of no return, so that she can climb off him and apply the squeeze. Once this part of the exercise is working, she remains sitting astride him, but now he thrusts gently until he can last for 15 minutes. Finally, they thrust simultaneously until he can last for 15 minutes.

Overcoming premature ejaculation on your own

Try the following exercises when you are alone:

- *masturbate with a dry hand until you can last for 15 minutes*

- *masturbate with a wet hand until you can last for 15 minutes.*

Remedies from the medicine cabinet

Doctors now think that as many as 60 percent of sex problems have physical causes.

Please pass the Viagra

Viagra is the recently developed drug treatment for impotence that helps a man gain and keep an erection. It has transformed the treatment of impotence by operating in two ways. First, it relaxes the muscles in the penis that allow blood to flow in and form a solid erection; second, it stimulates the brain to produce a certain reaction that tells the penis to become erect via erotic thoughts.

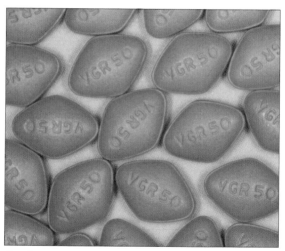

■ **Before you resort** *to Viagra to treat impotence, you should ensure that your relationship – as well as your body – is in good health.*

You need erotic thoughts for Viagra to work, so you genuinely have to desire your partner. And it isn't for everyone, as it can cause serious heart problems.

 Do not use Viagra without having a cardiac checkup first.

Viagra's predecessors

An earlier treatment for impotence involved injecting a drug into the penis. Although this method has been replaced by Viagra in the majority of cases, there are still some men for whom the injection method is a safer option. Supplements of the hormone testosterone may also be an effective alternative.

A certain percentage of men have a condition called "venous leakage." In these men, the blood that flows into the penis to form an erection almost immediately flows out again. Men who suffer from the condition often find that the simplest solution to the problem is a medically designed ring that fits around the base of the penis and keeps the blood in place. These rings are available from medical suppliers.

Slowing your guy down

Acute cases of premature ejaculation can be treated with a prescription drug called a beta-blocker, which lowers anxiety levels and slows down sexual response. Men already taking medication for heart problems must get professional medical advice.

Speeding your woman up

The drug phentolamine works on the "inhibitor" brain center by loosening up a person's inhibitions. This allows sexual desire to come to the surface.

 Do not take Viagra if you are a woman. No one knows yet what the side effects might be.

Some doctors prescribe the drug phentolamine as an aid to sexual arousal in women. A very few women are diagnosed as possessing low levels of the hormone testosterone, and testosterone replacement therapy may help.

Men and women who never feel sexy

The greatest sex problem today is low **libido**. You love your partner, but you just don't feel horny.

A low sex urge

If you possess virtually no sexual interest and never have done, there is a cocktail of hormones available to help you. These include testosterone and **DHEA**.

 Talk with your doctor about whether hormone supplements are right for you.

Different sex drives

If you and your partner have mismatched desires the following plan can help: you choose whether or not to have sex three days of the week, your partner chooses for the other three days of the week, and Sunday is up for grabs.

Your partner doesn't turn you on anymore

Try to get back in touch with each other using the sensate focus exercises that I described earlier in this chapter. Alternatively, it can help to talk things over with a relationship counselor.

What medicines are you taking?

There are a number of prescribed drugs that can kill sexual interest. These include some of the drugs for lowering blood pressure; some antihistamines in allergy medications, cold remedies, or travel sickness pills; some antidepressants and beta-blockers; too much estrogen; and major tranquilizers and sleeping preparations, such as barbiturates, taken for long periods. Even alternative therapies and natural supplements can have unwanted side effects.

 Don't stop taking medication suddenly. Consult your doctor first.

Life phases for men

Men experience less dramatic biological changes in life than women, yet the alterations are there, working away under the surface. Here is what men can expect.

Men: childhood and adolescence

Young male infants show explicit sexual responses. From birth boys experience regular erections, and they play with their genitals from the age of six months onward.

Puberty marks the start of interest in masturbation. If they are sexually active, boys of this age tend to be quick to reach arousal and orgasm, and quick to regain an erection.

Men: the 20s

Men usually try to become better lovers by learning about foreplay and exerting more control over ejaculation during intercourse as they get older. The early 20s are often spent enjoying the freedom associated with a single lifestyle, while the settling-down period tends to happen toward the end of the decade. Now, commitment becomes a major issue, and marriage and children may result.

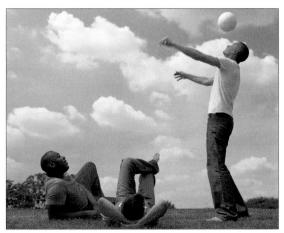

■ **The 20s** *are a transitional decade for men, and commitment to a partner may not yet be the priority.*

Men: the 30s and 40s

Relationships mature at this age, but sex can become routine. Overfamiliarity can lead to loss of interest in your partner. Men often deal with this by focusing more on a career or by developing a wandering eye.

 Unhealthy lifestyles can take their toll. Smoking, poor diet, stress, and obesity damage sexual performance.

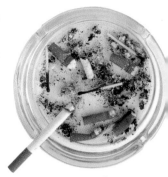

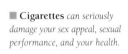 ■ **Cigarettes** *can seriously damage your sex appeal, sexual performance, and your health.*

The male hormone testosterone wanes extremely gradually from the mid-20s onward. As a result, men in their late 40s may notice that genital sensation is declining. Another symptom of low testosterone is mild depression. The collective name for symptoms caused by testosterone decline is andropause.

Men: the 50s and 60s

Aging brings a gradual decline in sex drive and ability. Nonetheless, the majority of men in this age bracket continue to want and enjoy sex, and they may discover that age brings several advantages.

 Men over 60 benefit from greater sexual experience, being less focused on penetration and orgasm, and taking longer to reach orgasm.

Men: over 70

Sex drive continues to decline slowly, and it becomes harder to sustain an erection. It also takes longer to regain the next erection, while ejaculation feels less powerful.

Life phases for women

Women experience many of the same sexual phases as men, but have some more obvious biological challenges.

Women: childhood and adolescence

Girls may start to play with their genitals at around ten months. After puberty, girls generally become interested in masturbation later than boys, and do it less frequently.

YOUR SEXUAL DIARY

The monthly rise and fall of hormones has a powerful effect on moods, well-being, and sexual sensitivity. Try keeping a daily diary in which you map your moods and physical feelings.

Women: the 20s and early 30s

Sexual knowledge and ability to reach orgasm increases with experience. As sex drive peaks during these decades, many women find that sex gets more enjoyable.

Having children can make an impact on a woman's sex life. Hormonal changes combined with the bodily changes brought about by childbirth can make some women feel less attractive. When added to the pressure of coping with a young child, this can cause sex drive to fly out the window.

■ **Having a baby** *inevitably has an impact on your lifestyle, and absorbs a great deal of time and energy.*

131

Women: the late 30s to early 40s

As children need less parenting, many women return to work or school and experience major personal growth. This can improve their sex lives by making them more confident. Alternatively, it may cause relationship problems if their partner is not keeping pace.

Women: the late 40s to 50s

The sexual effects of menopause differ from woman to woman. Some find that their sex drive diminishes, or that dryness and loss of orgasmic sensation turns them off. Others report that sex drive increases. Liberation from birth control makes some women footloose and fancy-free, while others feel less feminine and less sexy.

 Estrogen levels drop at menopause and this means that testosterone (which is responsible for sex drive) now has more impact.

Women: the 60s and over

Sexual enjoyment can continue indefinitely, just as long as general health remains good. Partners often find that the sexual effects of age – slow buildup, familiarity, and experience – can be used to their advantage.

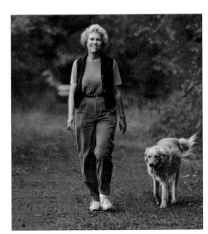

■ **Keeping fit** *as you grow older can help you to maintain and enjoy an active sex life.*

Getting professional help

When you've tried all the self-help techniques and nothing works, it's time to seek professional help.

Where to find a sex therapist

Big teaching hospitals often have sex therapy, psychiatric, and psychology departments. You may need a doctor's referral or you may be able to book yourself in directly. Most reputable sex therapists belong to professional organizations. See the Web sites resource section in the back of this book.

Is the therapist safe?

Most therapists give you intimate homework to do. There are, however, some therapists who specialize in doing physical work with their clients, but who state clearly before therapy begins that this is how they operate. This can mean doing physical exercises with your partner under the supervision of your therapist.

 No therapist should make personal sexual advances. If this happens, quit therapy at once.

Should you always see a doctor as well?

If you have any anxieties about your general or sexual health you should see a doctor. You may also need a doctor's referral for specialist consultations.

KEY POINTS
- *Sex problems are very common but they can usually be overcome using self-help techniques or, occasionally, prescribed drugs.*
- *Men and women go through sexual life stages. Understanding these stages can help to prevent and overcome problems.*
- *Sex therapy can help with intractable problems.*

Sexual dilemmas

SOMETIMES THINGS DON'T turn out as you would like them to. Sex may be fabulous, but you and your partner may fight all the time about showing affection. Or you may be passionate to an extreme, but your partner might not cope well with the intensity of your feelings. Perhaps you long to be close to the one you love, but when you achieve this you feel stressed by the experience. This chapter investigates a few of the dilemmas that show up in the bedroom.

Dilemmas of desire

More than 25 percent of young women don't always enjoy sex because intercourse brings them more pain than pleasure. Recently, a huge survey showed that two out of every five women and about one-third of men – in all age groups – experience some form of sexual dysfunction, ranging from lack of desire and attaining an erection to reaching orgasm. Here are some typical difficulties that sabotage good lovemaking.

When she wants it more than he does

Val always equated a good marriage with a lot of hot sex. She felt horny most of the time and would willingly have had sex at least once every day. Her partner, Alan, went along with this to begin with, but after about five months he felt deluged by sex. "I feel as if I am being forced to perform," Alan said.

Val, who had nothing but good intentions, felt terribly hurt by what she saw as Alan's rejection. "When he'd rather read than make love," she said, "I feel as if something is awfully wrong – with me."

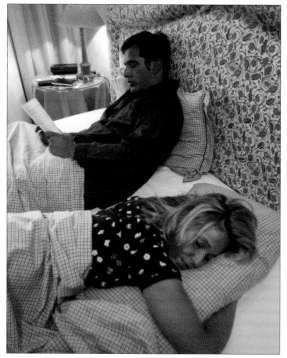

■ **Even if your partner** *would rather read in bed than make love, it does not necessarily mean that he or she is not in love with you.*

 Every individual has his or her own level of sexual desire, and sometimes these don't match up with a partner's.

Therapy helped Val understand that Alan's feelings had nothing to do with how lovable she was. In turn, Alan reassured her he loved her. But the couple also agreed to a sex contract, which took the pressure off them both.

 Making a sex contract – an agreement about the role sex plays in your lives together – can help ease tension in a relationship where one partner wants sex more often than the other.

135

When she is pregnant and he gets turned off

Bett was five months pregnant. She and her husband, Harvey, had planned this first child and were happy but Harvey seemed to have lost desire for his blossoming wife. And Bett was very unhappy. The sex act meant reassurance for her. Suddenly she was no longer able to feel that all was right with her world. And suppose Harvey never desired her again – even after the baby arrived?

Harvey's change of sexual desire is sadly common. Many men feel that the baby constitutes a third person present in bed and they become inhibited. Other men just don't find that fuller figure erotic. The solutions are long-term. Patience, a display of love and affection in place of sex, and massage, mutual masturbation, and oral sex can help. If the partnership doesn't recover once the baby's born, try focusing on sensate touch.

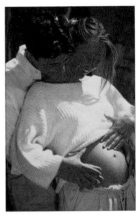

■ **For some people,** *a pregnant partner can be off-putting sexually. But don't despair: there are plenty of men who find the sight of a pregnant woman incomparably attractive.*

Sex positions for pregnancy

As pregnancy advances and your partner's breasts are tender and her belly swells, it's more comfortable to use either the woman-on-top position – if she still has the energy – or the side-by-side rear-entry position. The scissors position also works well, because the man's weight is not resting on her abdomen. In this position, he is on top, but lying across her thigh and to one side of her with one leg between hers and the other to the side; viewed from above, the couple forms a scissor-shape.

When he complains of losing sensation

Both men and women lose some sexual sensation as they age. Fifty-year-old Robert complained that he couldn't feel much during sex. His partner, Alison, complained that sex went on for hours.

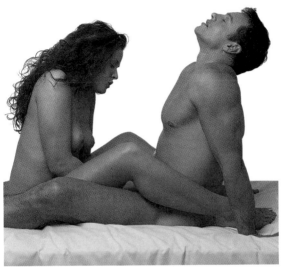

■ **Additional hand massage** *of the penis during intercourse increases the chances of orgasm for a man who has lost some sexual sensation. Extra stimulation can be enough to keep his erection and bring him to orgasm.*

Alison would be wise to help Robert's climax along by including hand massage with intercourse, or by bringing him close to orgasm before starting intercourse, or even by bringing him to orgasm after intercourse by hand alone. Other solutions might be hormones (testosterone and DHEA), which affect the whole sex hormone system, or Potency Plus, which stimulates the penis in particular.

 Older men generally need much more, and much stronger, sexual stimulation.

137

Intimacy issues

One of the biggest issues in the 21st century is that of commitment. Should we? Or shouldn't we?

When one person is not affectionate enough

Suzie complained that her man friend, Maurice, didn't kiss her enough. This mattered, she explained, because without kissing and intimate touching, she wasn't sure Maurice loved her. Suzie was 51, divorced, and had hoped that in Maurice she had found her next husband. But could she commit herself to someone who didn't feel quite right?

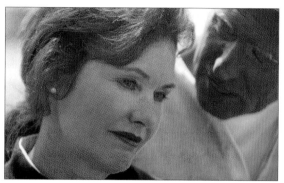

■ **Differences in the degree** *of affection that partners show each other can lead to an unhappy relationship. Talk these problems through.*

Maurice had grown up with unaffectionate parents. When he was a child, there had been no model of family affection to follow. But he did want Suzie. So he accepted that he needed to change. He rehearsed kissing and touching with Suzie and made certain he said "I love you" at least three times a week. His attempts meant a lot to Suzie because she could see that he cared enough to try. The relationship lasted.

In families where parents do not hug and kiss, the children don't learn how to engage in affectionate behavior.

Undemonstrative parents and children

Children of undemonstrative parents fail to make important brain connections about affection at the right age. So later in life, kissing and cuddling do not come naturally. Fortunately, warmth can still be learned.

When couples live physically apart

In this global age, many couples live in different houses or even countries, but remain committed to each other. One problem with this is that on the occasions when you are able to meet, it takes time to readjust to each other.

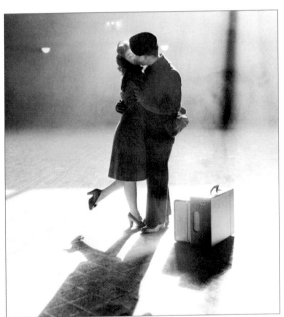

■ **The thrill of meeting** *your loved one for a special weekend together can be perpetual if you opt to live apart during the week.*

The solutions here tend to be practical ones. Usually one or both partners must readjust their working lives if they want the relationship to succeed. One partner might consider a transfer. Or the pattern of working could be adjusted; one partner might arrange telecommuting or flextime.

139

When one partner cannot commit

Rene was so overworked that he felt he didn't have time for marriage. But he did want a sex life. Julia, his girlfriend, who lived in her own apartment, understood his feelings to begin with, but found that, as time went by, she felt sidelined. She began to resent having sex with him and threatened to end things. He felt both saddened and pressured. Could there be a solution?

 Reluctance to commit is the relationship disease of our age.

Counseling helped Rene understand why Julia was upset. But Julia needed to feel valued by Rene, and some show of commitment was needed. She offered Rene three options.

1 *She could move in with him for a trial period with no strings attached.*

2 *They could get engaged, with a definite date for marriage and living together.*

3 *If he couldn't agree to either of these options, then the couple would separate.*

After some thought Rene agreed to the first option. A year later they were still together and agreed to start a family. Rene needed to move into intimacy at a pace where he felt he was in control. Julia had given him such an opportunity.

Balancing independence and intimacy

Couples find many ways of balancing their desire for sexual intimacy with their need for independence. Novelist Margaret Drabble lived in a separate home from her husband, the biographer Michael Ackroyd, for many years. Why should anyone want such a strange domestic setup? Perhaps someone felt cramped by parents as a child; in later life that person might need some space in order to be sincerely loving. Cohabiting might be associated with "doing one's duty" rather than loving spontaneously.

When one partner feels invaded

Kathryn had enjoyed a great sex life with her boyfriend, Frank, until he moved into her apartment. After a while, he complained that she was no longer interested in making love. She agreed, although she didn't understand why this should be. In counseling, the couple agreed that they loved each other and sincerely wanted the relationship to last. What could they do?

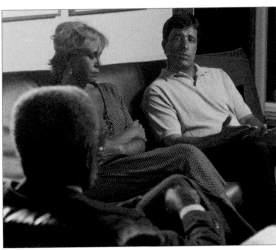

■ **Many couples may consider** *counseling as the last resort for their relationship. It can be revealing to get an outside perspective on the problem.*

Reclaiming some space

Kathryn discovered that she had felt invaded when Frank moved in. He had just assumed he was welcome and had declared his intentions instead of tactfully suggesting them. When Frank realized what he had done, he offered to move out so that the couple could reclaim their closeness. Instead the couple settled for sensate focusing and got back in touch with each other in unpressured circumstances. Frank's new insight into the problems of their relationship, plus the sensuality of regular touch, completely altered Kathryn's attitude and things improved greatly.

141

Strong feelings and your sex life

Anger, depression, anxiety, and mood swings can heighten or lower the amount of desire that you feel at any given time for your partner.

The rush that anger brings

Alice and Matt typically spent most evenings fighting, then making love. The problem was that after six years the fights had become more serious and Matt was getting turned off.

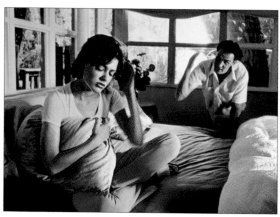

■ **Try not to let** *arguments and make-up sex become a regular occurrence, as they can turn into an integral part of your relationship.*

Alice realized that her reason for picking fights was boredom. Their first move to remedy the problem was to make a peace pact. Their second move was to develop a joint project so that sex was no longer their sole stimulus. The plan worked well. A year later they were calmer and more stable.

Moods swings: the ups and downs of PMS

David never knew where he stood with his girlfriend, Caroline. Sometimes she couldn't drag him into the bedroom often enough; then for several days at a time she would have nothing to do with him. David was beginning to have serious doubts about Caroline.

Coping with PMS

A visit to a counselor established that Caroline had bad PMS, which made her withdrawn in the days before her period. Once David understood that her behavior was, to some extent, predictable, he felt sympathetic. Caroline also changed the type of contraceptive pill she was taking and her mood swings evened out.

The black cloud of depression

Maria had tried everything to get Julio interested in her sexually again, but nothing was working. In counseling Julio revealed that he was desperately worried about his family business. If the business failed several close relations would be out of work.

 Extreme stress and depression can actually depress the sex urge; depression lowers levels of testosterone.

When Maria understood that Julio was too anxious to have sex she became extremely supportive. The crisis eventually lifted and, thanks to Maria's patience, their sex life came back.

The green-eyed monster

Polly couldn't cope with the fact that her husband Victor had always been a flirt and became convinced he was having an affair. She responded by embarking upon a "revenge affair" herself. "It made me feel better – for a short time. But then I began to feel guilty. I'm not sure now that Victor was sleeping around."

Even if Victor was not having an affair, he was always putting Polly down and he made her feel inferior in bed. Polly decided to confront him every single time he was rude, regardless of the circumstances. This was tough to start with, but actually improved the relationship in the long term.

Medical minefields

Many people take drugs for legitimate medical reasons, but find that they are cursed with undesirable sexual side effects. It is important for you to know that certain medications carry a risk. And you should always tell your doctor if you have problems with impotence, loss of desire, vaginal dryness, inability to achieve orgasm, or problems with ejaculation. Many people suffer from feelings of shame and inadequacy about their sex problems. Knowing that their medication is to blame can help them avoid emotional problems as well.

Don't let embarrassment keep you from consulting your doctor about sexual problems.

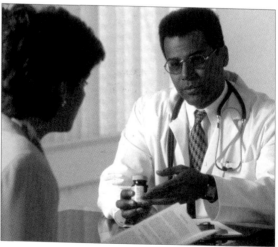
■ **Your doctor** *should be willing to answer queries you might have about whether your prescription could have a negative influence on your sex life.*

How medication can affect sex

The following table summarizes some of the major classes of medication and the sexual problems associated with them. Do bear in mind, however, that some drugs may only cause problems when they are combined with alcohol or other drugs.

SEX AND DRUGS

Antidepressants

Monoamine oxidase inhibitors (MAOIs), including pargyline hydrochloride, phenelzine (Nardil), nialamide May cause sexual problems for a small percentage of users. Some women may find they decrease sexual desire and make it harder to reach orgasm. Men may find they cause erection problems or delayed ejaculation.

Tricyclics, including clomipramine hydrochloride (Anafranil) Depression itself causes loss of desire, so recovery through treatment can alleviate this. Some people taking tricyclics, however, find that they decrease sex drive. May cause erection and ejaculation problems for men and problems reaching orgasm for women.

Fluoxetine hydrochloride (Prozac) High percentage of users find it harder to ejaculate or achieve orgasm.

Antihistamines

Histamine H1-receptor antagonists in motion sickness, hay fever, and cough remedies, including diphenhydramine hydrochloride (Benadryl, Benylin). Sexual desire may be reduced; causes vaginal dryness in some women.

Histamine H2-receptor antagonists in ulcer and heartburn treatments, including cimetidine (Tagamet). Sexual desire may be reduced; causes erection problems for some men.

Anti-Parkinson drugs

L-dopa (including Larodopa) Sexual desire may increase.

Cholesterol-lowering drugs

Clofibrate (Atromid-S) Sexual desire may be reduced; causes erection problems for some men.

SEX AND DRUGS

Blood-pressure control (hypertension) drugs

Centrally-acting drugs, including methyldopa (Aldomet, Dopamet). High doses can decrease desire; erection and ejaculation problems for men; orgasm problems for women.

Alpha-blockers, including prazosin hydrochloride (Minipress); beta-blockers, including propanolol hydrochloride; vasodilators, including hydralazine hydrochloride. May reduce sexual desire; may cause erection problems in men.

Diuretics

Thiazides, including bendroflumethiazide (Naturetin). For a small percentage of users, desire may be reduced; women may experience vaginal dryness; and men may suffer erection problems.

Loop diuretics, e.g., frusemide; potassium-sparing diuretics, e.g., spironolcatone. High dosages can cause reduction in sexual desire. Women may experience vaginal dryness; men may suffer erection problems.

Hormonal preparations

Anabolic steroids, including nandrolone, stanozolol. Misuse causes serious problems. In men, testosterone levels may drop, resulting in loss of sex drive, shrinkage of testicles, damaged sperm production, and enlargement of the breasts. Women risk developing masculine characteristics (facial and body hair, male-pattern baldness), menstrual and ovulation problems, and enlargement of the clitoris. Rapid mood swings, rages, and even psychosis can also result.

Androgens, such as testosterone preparations. May help to restore sex drive and orgasmic ability to men and women. High doses can cause problems: development of masculine features in women; impaired sperm production in men.

Anti-androgens May reduce sexual desire in both men and women. May cause erection and ejaculation problems and impaired sperm production.

Estrogens May improve vaginal lubrication in postmenopausal women, but may cause loss of sex drive and serious erection and ejaculation problems in men.

Oral contraceptives Women have extremely variable reactions; sex drive may increase or decrease.

Sleeping preparations

Barbiturates Addiction and long-term use may cause loss of sex drive in women and erection problems in men.

Nonbarbiturates Sexual side effects are rare.

Tranquilizers

Benzodiazepines, including lorazepam (Ativan), chlordiazepoxide (Librium), diazepam (Valium), clorazepate dipotassium (Tranxene). May reduce sexual desire. May cause erection problems for men; orgasm problems for women.

Phenothiazines, including chlorpromazine hydrochloride (Thorazine, Largactil); butyrophenones, including benperidol. Sexual desire is often reduced; some men may experience ejaculation problems; high doses may cause erection problems.

KEY POINTS

- Sometimes sex is hampered by different levels of desire between partners.
- Intimacy and commitment issues can affect the quality of your sex life.
- Powerful emotions such as anger or jealousy can damage your sex drive.
- Some prescribed drugs can have a negative effect on your sex drive.

Glossary

Clitoris
A small and elongated organ toward the front of the vulva that is highly sensitive. Stimulating this erectile organ provides women with great pleasure.

Desensitization technique
Many lovers are turned on by dirty talk, but are too shy to try it. This technique helps to alleviate shyness by desensitizing you or your lover to the words you feel most bashful about. This is done by reading out a list of these words in front of a mirror until you can say them without cringing. Practicing this technique with your partner can also be funny, and humor is an excellent desensitizing tool.

DHEA
Dehydroepiandrosterone (DHEA) is a hormone produced by the adrenal gland. Low levels of DHEA are associated with low sex drive. It is thought that high levels of stress may cause an imbalance of DHEA. Supplements can increase sex drive.

Erogenous zones
These are areas of the body that are sensitive to stimulation. Some are common to most people, such as the lips and nipples, while others are more unusual. Getting to know each other's erogenous zones, and the type of touch that arouses each one, is a very pleasurable way of developing intimacy.

Fetishes
When someone has a fetish, they are highly aroused by handling a particular object or part of the body that is not a sexual organ. For example, some people are very turned on by feet (known as foot fetishists) while others are driven to distraction by the smell and texture of rubber. Fetishes can be used to highten sexual arousal and satisfaction.

Genitals
The sexual organs – the penis and testicles in men, and the labia, clitoris, and vagina in women.

Kama Sutra
An ancient Indian text on erotic pleasure within marriage. This well-respected font of fascinating knowledge is one of the oldest sex manuals in the world.

Labia
The labia are the folds of skin surrounding and protecting the vagina and

clitoris, consisting of the labia minora (the inner two folds of skin) and the labia majora (the outer two folds).

Libido
Your libido is your sex drive. Some people have a very robust libido, while others have a much less demanding one. With most people, libido can be greatly affected by both mood and stress levels.

Petting
Kissing and caressing erotically is known as petting.

Prostate gland
A gland found in the male body, close to the bladder and urethra. It secrets seminal fluid. Stimulating the prostate via the anus can be highly arousing for many men.

Pubococcygeal (PC) muscle
This muscle (also known as the pelvic floor) holds the pelvic organs within the pelvic region. It is the muscle that you squeeze when you want to stop the flow of urine. A woman squeezing the PC muscle during sex can give her man, and herself, extra sensation. For men, PC muscle exercises can help to maintain an erection.

Sensate focus exercises
These exercises are designed to help couples learn about one another's – and their own – sexual responses to stimulation. They can be very helpful in a sexual relationship in which you feel as if you have got off on the wrong foot, or got stuck in a rut, as they can help you discover (or rediscover) how to arouse one another.

Sexologists
People who study the sexual behavior of humans.

Sexual biographies
Your sexual biography is everything that has contributed to your sexual nature, including experiences, education, impressions, and religious upbringing and attitudes.

Urethra
The channel or "tube" that takes urine from the bladder and out of the body. In men, this channel also acts as a channel for ejecting semen.

Virgin
A person who has never had penetrative sex is known as a virgin.

Index

Acknowledgments

Dorling Kindersley would like to thank the following people for their contributions during the creation of this book.

Picture researchers: Carlo Ortu, Samantha Nunn.

Picture librarians: Romaine Werblow, Claire Bowers.

Indexer: Hilary Bird.

Proofreader: Constance Novis.

The publisher would also like to thank all the models who appear in the book.

Picture Credits

0 Corbis: Jennie Woodcock; Reflections Photolibrary; 8 www.bridgeman.co.uk: Musee Rodin, Paris, France -9; 10 Getty Images: Bruce Ayres b.; 13 Corbis: Todd Haimann b.; 28 Mary Evans Picture Library: b.; 29 Moviestore Collection: cl.; 30 Moviestore Collection: c.; 32 Getty Images: Klaus Lahnstein c.; 34 Getty Images: John Lamb b.; 37 Getty Images: Lonnie Duka cb.; 38 Getty Images: Karen Beard cfl.; 40 Moviestore Collection: b.; 60 ImageState/Pictor: The Slide File -61.; 83 Corbis: Richard T. Nowitz cb.; 92 Getty Images: Jerome Tisne b.; 94 Photonica: Bunni Lezak ca.; 95 Getty Images: Alan Becker br.; 96 Zefa Visual Media: masterfile / Kevin Dodge b.; 97 Getty Images: Sean Murphy b.; 98 Getty Images: Barbara Peacock b.; 99 Getty Images: Alberto Incrocci b.; 100 Getty Images: Bart Geerligs cra.; 101 Corbis: Ed Kashi ca.; 102 Corbis: -103.; 115 Corbis: Michael Pole t.; 116 Katz/FSP: Simon Grosset crb.; 117 Corbis: PN016962 c.; 118 Corbis: Earl & Nazima Kowall cfr.; 121 Corbis: Niall Benvie c.; 122 ImageState /Pictor: AGE Fotostock c.; 126 Science Photo Library: John Greim b.; 129 Getty Images: Jason Hetherington b.; 132 Getty Images: Benn & Esther Mitchell b.; 135 Getty Images: Michelangelo Gratton t.; 136 Getty Images: Laurence Monneret cfr.; 138 Getty Images: David Hanover c.; 139 Corbis: Bettmann c.; 141 Getty Images: Zigy Kaluzny c.; 142 Getty Images: Rick Rusing c.; 144 Corbis: John Henley c.

All other images © Dorling Kindersley. For further information see: www.dkimages.com